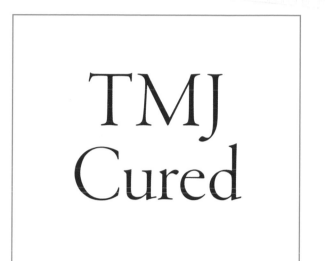

TMJ
Cured

TMJ
Cured

Fixing the Bite Is the Answer

Philip L. Taylor, DDS

TRUTH IN DENTISTRY PUBLISHING
Palm Desert, California

First printing 2010

ISBN 978-0-9823910-0-6
LCCN 2009927847

ATTENTION CORPORATIONS, UNIVERSITIES, COLLEGES, AND PROFESSIONAL ORGANIZATIONS: Quantity discounts are available on bulk purchases of this book for educational, gift purposes, or as premiums for increasing magazine subscriptions or renewals. Special books or book excerpts can also be created to fit specific needs. For information, please contact Truth In Dentistry Publishing, 72937 Willow Street, Palm Desert, CA 92260; 760-469-3579; www.tmjcured.com.

CONTENTS

FOREWORD

"TEACHER" DOES NOT describe Dr. Philip Taylor accurately although he is one of the finest I have ever met. Neither does "Professor" although he has been on the faculty at the USC School of Dentistry for many years. While each title connotes the dispensing of information, admittedly at different levels of sophistication, they both fall short of the mark—his mark. It is in Italian that we find a more appropriate moniker for this special man: *maestro*, one who has truly mastered his craft and now illuminates the path for others to follow. Dr. Taylor's career has taken him on a journey of discovery and assimilation as his acumen and expertise have increased from pedodontics to restorative dentistry to orthodontics to organic occlusion (gnathology). Ever a student of the profession, he has doggedly persisted in finding answers to his patients' TM joint and bite problems. He has associated with and has been mentored by the giants of gnathology, resulting in his becoming (in the minds of many) one of them.

Nature has an ingenious way of creating functional harmony, even out of chaos—for a while. The body's adaptive capabilities can tolerate a bite that is "off" and have it masquerade as normal—for a while. Anatomy, physiology, gender, diet, stress, and dental treatment (the list goes on) can all play a role in challenging that alleged state of harmony. Time is often the precipitating agent in causing these diverse influences to conjoin and then create symptoms. I tell my younger adult patients that they are "bullet proof" until the age of thirty. Then they will have to work hard to stay healthy when before it just came naturally.

The body (bite) will only take so much abuse before it begins to rebel. And as Dr. Taylor so eloquently chronicles in this book, that rebellion (symptoms) does not always confine itself to the teeth. This ability for the body to adapt is both patients' best friend and their worst enemy. Because there are no obvious problems, most dentists become "tooth doctors," limiting their practices to treating one or two teeth at a time. They ask the patient to bite down on a new restoration, and as long as it isn't high (hyper-occlusion), they assume the body will adapt to any minor irregularities in the bite. To their credit most dentists do this very well. To their discredit there is a lot more going on. Some don't know any better. Some don't care. Dr. Taylor knows and cares—hence, the genesis of this book.

Treating dental disease is much more than just ensuring teeth are free from decay. It is about creating harmony within the entire stomatognathic system: teeth, gums (periodontium), temporomandibular joint (TM joint), and muscles. Leave any one out of the equation, and it's like baking a cake, halving the sugar, and then wondering why it's not quite like mom's. It looks like cake, it smells like cake, it's edible, it's acceptable (to some)—just not as good as you-know-who used to make. You get the idea. The teeth are a set of gears anchored in bone surrounded by gum tissue. The upper and lower jaws are attached to each other by the most complex joint in the entire body, the

TM joint. Powerful muscles guide and direct the movement of the lower jaw, allowing the teeth (gears) to do their jobs of chewing and speaking. If the TM joint and the teeth are not in sync, those muscles can literally destroy an otherwise healthy dentition, even one completely free of decay!

And we're not talking about just a few people. The bad news is that this condition is pandemic. It is estimated that 95 percent of the population has a bite problem! The good news is that of those who develop symptoms, 95 percent can be treated successfully.

This condition lurks silently like a sleeping dragon, a malevolent beast, waiting for the right conditions to stir it from its slumber and wreak havoc among an unsuspecting public and, dare I say, profession. These patients need a white knight like Dr. Taylor and those like him who are trained to slay this dragon or at least tame it and put it back into its lair, to restore homeostasis to a stressed stomatognathic system that the body (nature) is no longer able to cope with. I rest my case.

In this book Dr. Taylor documents for the patient and practitioner the rationale behind and the evidence for successful TM joint therapy. When Bill Clinton was running for office, it was James Carville who kept reminding the public, "It's the economy, stupid!" When it comes to treating TM joint dysfunction, Dr. Taylor keeps reminding us, "It's the bite, ladies and gentlemen!" We live in the "information age." Consumers have access to educational materials enabling them to ask more intelligent questions regarding their health and treatment options. The information contained in this book gives the public the tools to help find those clinicians sufficiently trained to treat TMJ. It is poignant, I think, that Dr. Taylor calls out to his colleagues to become one of them.

When the day is done and the race has been run, most people will be inclined to ask the following, "Have I left this world a little better having lived my life?" As I look back over Dr. Taylor's career, the many, many patients he has helped when no one else could, the many students he has taught and continues to teach, his generosity in mentoring anyone serious about improving his or her professional skills, I believe I can answer for him. Those of us fortunate enough to have known Phil would in chorus resoundingly reply, "*Yes!*"

I know you are going to enjoy reading this book. It is my sincerest wish that the information contained within will help you obtain a less stressful and healthier life.

—*John J. Petrini, DDS*

The Most Underutilized Dental Treatment

THE ACRONYM TMJ stands for "temporomandibular joint," which is the jaw joint where the jaw hinges and translates. In this book I use TMJ to refer to the disease, not the jaw joint itself, as that has become common usage. Technically, we should use the acronym TMD or TMJD, which means "temporomandibular dysfunction" (or disease). People say, "I have TMJ," and they mean they have the disease, not the jaw joint. In order to be clear, I will write "TM joint" when I'm talking about the jaw joint and will reserve "TMJ" for the disease.

In junior high school I took woodshop, metal shop, and general science. I loved building boats and all kinds of woodwork, and I won a few awards. I remember watching a couple of friends of mine trying to drive a nail into a board. It was so strange to watch because they seemed so clumsy. Maybe I began to realize I had some mechanical abilities and needed to put them to good use. I came from a mechanical family. My father was a graduate of New York University with a degree in mechanical engineering. He became a pilot in the First World War and then taught auto shop in high school. He worked his way up teaching mechanical drawing, then mathematics, and became the high school principal. My older brother was a graduate of Cal Tech and worked for Northrop Aircraft for a lifetime. So when I started pre-med at College of Pacific and lived with some pre-dental students, I became increasingly aware of how dentists use their hands and shifted my interest to dentistry.

IN ORDER TO BE CLEAR, I WILL WRITE "TM JOINT" WHEN I'M TALKING ABOUT THE JAW JOINT AND WILL RESERVE "TMJ" FOR THE DISEASE.

In 1950 my practice began in San Diego, with a second office in El Cajon. Then I worked full-time in El Cajon, where I built a two-story building that had ten suites to rent and my own office with five chairs and a lab. About a decade later I traveled to USC Dental School to teach one day a week and found the direction I had to go as I learned more than I taught. The principles I now love teaching, which were not taught in my undergraduate experience, came from those five years at USC. What really finalized and solidified my understanding that correcting the bite always comes first (before all other dental procedures) was joining the Gus Swab study club in 1979.

When I started to use this bite correction procedure, I had no idea of the possibilities. I believed all I had to focus on was saving teeth and gums from destruction. After about twenty-three years of practice, I found that I needed to know more in order to do certain things like TMJ. Then I began to learn from the masters about "gnathology," the science of the jaws. These teachings concern the engineering principles involving the movements of the jaw.

If a person's teeth come together properly when chewing, speaking, swallowing, or just biting off a thread, then the jaw, like any mechanical device, would not wear out. But since the jaw does wear out, I proceeded to correct peoples' bites. At first the cases were limited to patients without very many teeth. I found that the appliances they wore prior to my correction of the bite never worked or were uncomfortable. Then, when I had finished, they told me they felt a huge difference. They explained that the artificial teeth I had made felt right. There was no feeling that the appliance was artificial.

Then I began to correct the bite of folks who had all their teeth because the procedure was becoming second nature now. The reports of all sorts of ailments disappearing after this procedure rocked my dental mindset because none of these ailments was directly connected at all with the teeth. So my instincts told me that the jaw joint must have nerves that connected with other nerves all over the body. Since this joint or actually these joints—because there are two of them—are so close to the brain, ears, eyes, and balancing mechanism, the posture of the seated lower jaw in its socket means a whole lot more than we thought it did. This discovery changed my whole practice.

Dizzy spells, ringing in the ears, headaches, pains, and strange noises in the head may all be attributable to poor posture in the joint.

The seated posture of the lower jaw in its socket when the teeth are fully closed together may be either good or not-so-good. When the teeth are straightened or filed upon, worn down, capped, or even filled, the bite can change, thereby changing the jaw joint posture. Dentists are often then called upon to change the bite back to the original position or to create a new good bite.

Oddly but tellingly, except for the bite on full dentures (plates), I didn't know what a good bite was—and I had been practicing dentistry for twenty-eight years. Fortunately, human beings have a great capacity to adapt to different inaccuracies of the bite, so dentists get by without too many complaints. Still, we can do better.

My book covers the following topics: first, the need for better dental education about the occlusion; second, the correction technique itself and the controversies surrounding it; and, third, some of the historical background behind the controversy. My thesis is that dentists must strive to improve their knowledge and learn the technique called "occlusal correction" and that patients need to be more aware of what it can do to alleviate their problems.

I believe that occlusal correction is the most underutilized procedure in dentistry today. Think of the thousands of dental offices that need to utilize this revolutionary technique before a bridge, partial denture, or implant is made. One thing for sure we know—this bite correction procedure should always be done prior to any TMJ work, any periodontal work, and any major reconstruction work.

I BELIEVE THAT OCCLUSAL CORRECTION IS THE MOST UNDERUTILIZED PROCEDURE IN DENTISTRY TODAY.

Perhaps you are wondering, where am I going to find a dentist trained to change my bite? Our organization is called the International Academy of Gnathology and is found on the Internet (www.gnathologyusa.org/). Its members are the dentists who are interested in the principles of bite engineering. Most are dentists who think outside the box and can help you.

When you talk to a prospective dentist to do your occlusal correction, first ask whether he or she knows what organic occlusion is. If you get the right answer, then talk to one of his or her cured TMJ patients.

CHAPTER 1

TMJ
and Its Causes

AS NOTED PREVIOUSLY, there are actually two TM joints, one on either side of the face, located just in front of the ear. They are complex joints because they have two compartments, an upper where the jaw slides and a lower where the jaw hinges. (See figure 1.)

TWO COMPARTMENTS IN TM JOINT

The compartments are separated by a disc, which is held in place by ligaments and muscles. It separates the bones of the joint, the mandible (or lower jaw), and the skull (or cranium). The temporal bone that forms the upper half of the TM joint houses the "glenoid fossa," which has the thickest and strongest bone just above and slightly forward of the head of the "condyle." This thick part continues forward and becomes the "articular tubercle." The "articular disc" is pulled forward with the condyle head as the jaw goes forward and downward to incise. There is a stretchable ligament at the rear of the disc to bring it back when the jaw is returned. Notice the "synovial

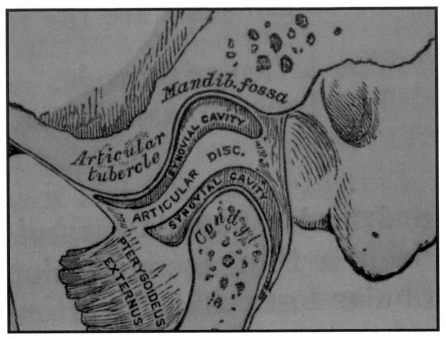

FIGURE 1: *Sagittal section through the TM joint*
In this illustration the teeth are to the left and the ear opening to the right.

cavity" between the bone above and the disc below. This cavity is where the slide takes place. The "synovial cavity" below the disc is where the rotation or opening and closing of the mandible takes place.

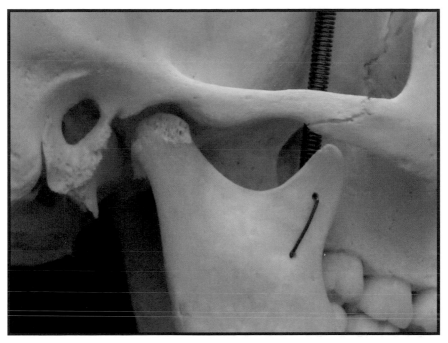

FIGURE 2: *The TM joint in a skull without muscles and ligaments*
Notice in figure 2 the space between the "condyle" and the "fossa," which
houses the "disc" and its ligaments.

The muscle that attaches to the front of the articular disc
is called the "lateral pterygoid" and is attached to the "condyle"
also. Then there is a ligament that stretches like elastic to pull
the disc back as the bone returns to the socket to chew. This
disc is similar to the ones in between our vertebrae. The temporal bone is shaped like a socket with a ramp on the front
("eminence") for the mandible to slide down when it comes
forward to incise or bite off a carrot. The purpose of this ramp
is to create separation for the back part of the jaw so the gears
(cusps) on the back teeth won't clash and wear out. The front
teeth at the forward end of the mandible separate the front
chewing teeth so they don't wear out when the jaw comes forward to incise.

THE ANGLE OF THE EMINENCE

Imagine for a moment that the "eminence" or ramp of the jaw was flat instead of about a 45-degree angle, so that the condyle traveled straight forward instead of downward. This arrangement would not allow the back end of the mandible to separate the cusps of the back teeth. Notice in the next illustration (figure 3) how the model shows the mandible sliding forward and all teeth are separating due to the ramp ("eminence") in the TM joint and the slope of the backs of the upper front teeth.

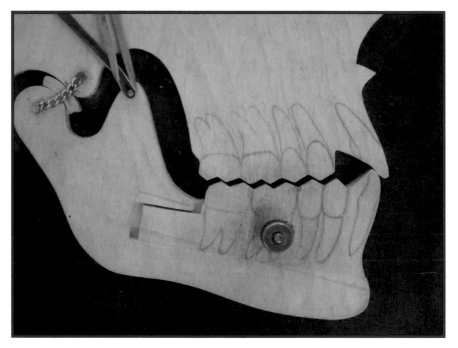

FIGURE 3: *Model of the jaws and TM joint*

Notice the small gold chain in the TM joint. It represents the ligaments that hold the jaw from going backward but allow it to go forward. If the jaw was pushed back, the chain (ligaments) would tighten and limit the backward travel. The teeth separate as the jaw moves forward (to the right) because the lower front teeth slide down the backs of the upper front teeth. The condyle slides down the eminence to separate the back teeth. The angle of "eminence" and the angle of the "backs of the upper front teeth" must be greater than the steepness of the cusps; otherwise, the teeth would interfere with and wear or clash with each other.

ANATOMY

Let's look at the ligaments in the joint itself. This picture (figure 4) is from *Gray's Anatomy*, showing the mandible and the cranium with the condyle encased in the capsular ligament and the temporomandibular ligament. Notice that the ligaments prevent the condyle from traveling backward toward the ear opening. There is no stretch to these ligaments. If a dentist were

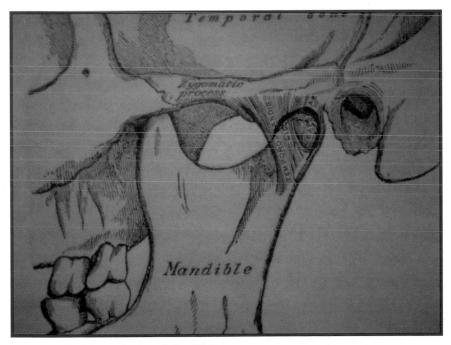

FIGURE 4: *Ligaments of the TM joint*

to push back on the mandible to seat it in the rearmost position, to find out where the teeth came together in that position, the condyle would seat not farther back but rotate upward due to the ligaments. This is an important consideration for organic occlusion, which will be discussed in chapter 3.

The disc is limited from traveling sideways by the capsular ligaments attached to the poles of the condyle, much the same as a skull cap loosely attached to your ears would work. You could pull the cap forward and back on your head, but it couldn't slip off sideways. The idea of the front muscle and the rear ligament is to keep the disc in the best possible position in order to separate the bones and provide a cushion effect. Because of the complexity of this double joint we still don't know everything we need to know about it. What we do know about it is that when the torque produced by missing teeth, misplaced teeth, or dental work not in harmony with the existing bite is corrected, the joint has the best chance to heal. This undue stress on the joint should always be corrected first when treating TMJ. My favorite easy explanation of TMJ is summarized by asking: "If you sprained your ankle, would you go to the doctor wearing high-heeled shoes?" (The heels represent the wrong bite.) And a follow-up question might be: "Do I need surgery, or shall I just wear flats?"

THIS UNDUE STRESS ON THE JOINT SHOULD ALWAYS BE CORRECTED FIRST WHEN TREATING TMJ.

SYMPTOMS

Symptoms of TMJ are numerous and confusing. It is confusing because TMJ mimics many other diseases. It can be confused with: 1) sinus infection; 2) ear, mastoid infections, and Ménière's disease; 3) tooth infections and pathology; 4) a variety of lesser occurring diseases like arthritis. Once these other problems are ruled out, we can begin to diagnose TMJ. Most of my patients who seek my help already know they have TMJ. These symptoms I have listed below come from patients I have treated and are probably not all of the many different symptoms of TMJ.

HEADACHES

Headaches are probably one of the most common symptoms of TMJ. They can be divided into types by names such as migraine, tension, cluster, and a few others. Restoring the bite to organic occlusion relieves most of these problems if they originated with the bite.

HEADACHES ARE PROBABLY ONE OF THE MOST COMMON SYMPTOMS OF TMJ.

Example of a Headache

One of the most dramatic cases of a headache attributable to TMJ came from my practice in El Cajon. The patient had lost a tooth in an accident and needed to have it replaced with bridgework. I explained that I needed to correct the bite before the replacement was attempted. The patient asked whether that procedure could help her headaches, and I said yes. We completed the correction in one appointment, and she walked out of the office in disbelief. The headache she had coming in was gone while she was in the chair. The "cure" lasted about a week; then, she was back. A small correction, taking about half an hour, produced the same result. She was so impressed (and so was I) that she was free from migraines that she went dancing that night. Her migraines had caused her agony and required injections of Demerol over the previous twenty years. She had tried everything, including acupuncture, which only helped while she was being treated. Her TMJ healed and shifted her bite, causing probably six to eight more minor corrections, each with the delightful result of freedom from a headache. She went on a trip overseas for the first time in years because of the freedom from headaches. While on this trip, her headache returned, and she begged and borrowed pills from her fellow travelers until she could get home to call me. A minor correction was all it took. The last time she called me was nearly a year later. I heard this voice on the phone that sounded like someone talking with clenched teeth. She had muscle spasms that wouldn't allow her full opening of her jaws. I successfully corrected the bite again with the same miraculous result.

PAINS

Pain in a variety of places is probably the next most common symptom of TMJ. The pain can be very obvious in the joints, near by them or it can be far removed from the joints. Anywhere in the head or neck is a frequent location. It can be in or around the teeth and jaws. Sometimes the patient is certain he or she has a toothache from a cavity or a cracked tooth. These cases can be difficult to diagnose. I've had patients certain that they were about to lose a tooth from an abscess only to find that the bite was too high on that particular tooth.

PHANTOM TOOTHACHE

"Phantom" toothache is the name for this phenomenon. I can remember a tooth that was bothering a patient when the

X-rays showed nothing and vitality tests proved negative. I assured the patient there was nothing I could find wrong. She kept complaining to the point that I referred her to an endodontist, who couldn't find any problem either. He finally did a root canal on the tooth, but the pain in it persisted. One of the routine treatments after the root canal is to grind down the surface of the tooth to prevent a fracture since the non-vital tooth is more brittle. When this was done, the pain suddenly left.

MUSCLE PAIN

Muscle pain probably is the most common type that we encounter. It can vary from severe to mild. The muscles that perform the chewing motion are the ones most often involved. The neighboring neck, shoulder, chest, and back muscles are sometimes involved also. Generally, we can have the patient point to the source of the pain and find tenderness there.

MYOFASCIAL PAIN DYSFUNCTION

Muscle pain derived from TM joints is often referred to as MPD or myofascial pain dysfunction. This term is used to separate a muscle disorder from a joint disorder.

TIC-DOULOUREUX

I have had several cases of tic-douloureux or trigeminal neuralgia that might fall into the TMJ category.

An Example of Tic-douloureux

One case I encountered was so severe that the patient considered suicide. He was referred to me by his physician after more than ten years of suffering. He had a severe shooting pain down the right side of his lower jaw. It would start with little twitches of pain, itches or tingling that would give him warning that the major, intense "bolt of lightning" pain was coming. He would have to stop what he was doing because of the severity of it. If he was eating, he would stop and get up and go into a room by himself and try to deal with it. The attacks would occur about once every hour. They would last about two to three minutes. The severity of the pain on a scale of 1 to 10, 10 being the most severe, he stated was a 12. He sought help from everyone he could think of. When I saw him, I made my routine examination with mounted models and X-rays. He had many kinds of dentistry from silver amalgam fillings, gold in-lays, porcelain over metal crowns, and plastic fillings. My first recommendation was to correct his bite, then secondarily, if this didn't help, to restore his dental work to all of some type of non-metal restoration so that there wouldn't be any electrical disturbances. After a simple but accurate occlusal correction, his pain vanished and hasn't recurred in thirteen years last I heard. I have a video of this man's testimony; it was such a dramatic cure.

An Example of Pain from a Cross-Bite Malocclusion

Another patient suffering from a strange type of pain had a cross-bite on her right side in the cuspid area that caused her jaw, when fully closed, to deviate to her right. After I corrected this bite problem, the pain in her chest wall disappeared. This pain had centered somewhere in the middle of her right chest. She described it as halfway forward from her right scapula. Her physicians tried everything, including injecting Novocain deep into her chest cavity. They succeeded in numbing the entire chest but didn't stop the pain. This no doubt was a true referred pain from the TM joints. Her MRIs showed that the discs between the bones of the TM joints were completely gone or non-functional. Bone was rubbing on bone with no complaints about her TM joints. All I did was correct her bite, and the pain in her chest vanished. Her case, however, required about seven years of follow-up adjustments because of the severe disfigurement of the joint mechanisms. She had many setbacks, but each one responded to a very accurate adjustment back to organic occlusion. Even though she had severe joint damage, the occlusal correction renewed the freedom of joint torque so she could continue to heal. Each time I adjusted her back to organic occlusion, she was free of pain.

One of the symptoms of the need for an adjustment was a feeling of extreme exhaustion. When the patient walked out twenty-five minutes later, her total strength and energy were restored.

DIGESTION

I've had some digestive track problems clear up after correction of the bite. One case that was illustrative of this was an elderly lady I had taken care of for many years. She finally gave in to my nagging about her bite and allowed me to correct it. When I had finished and allowed time for the retreat, healing, and deteriorated dentistry replacement, she confessed that her constipation had disappeared.

EARS

Dizzy spells, Ménière's disease, and ringing in the ears can also be related to problems with the bite. In one such extreme case the patient was so dizzy she couldn't get out of bed and suffered also from nausea and loss of hearing. When she could come to my office, I found that orthodontics was necessary to overcome and correct her gross overjet problem.

"Overjet" means the horizontal distance between the upper and lower front teeth. The slang for "overjet" is "buck teeth." This problem disallows proper disclusion or separation of the gearing of the back teeth and produces a strain on the TM joints.

My patient's symptoms gradually subsided as the bite and engineering of her jaws changed.

MÉNIÈRE'S DISEASE

Ringing in the ears and dizziness can come from other sources (such as high blood pressure), but I have been successful in treating about half the cases referred to me. There can, though, be inner ear disturbances that need careful attention by experts, such as "the House Clinic" in the Los Angeles area.

Ménière's disease is usually the diagnosis when these kinds of ear problems occur. It is located in the inner ear and is blamed on excessive fluid or fluid balance. The recommended treatment has to do with eliminating salt and dietary controls. Often tubes are placed to drain the fluid and relieve the pressure. Burt Reynolds had this done and gained relief from his dizzy spells. His story will be told later.

Weakness and exhaustion that is unexplained can also have its origin in the TM joints. I've had several cases that were dramatically improved in just a few minutes with occlusal adjustments.

EYESIGHT

Problems with eyesight can be connected to the TM joints. I had an electrician patient who after the correction got up out of the chair, took off his glasses, and exclaimed, "It's like I took off a pair of smoky glasses—everything is clear—the greens are greener and blues are bluer." He was overjoyed. When he returned for follow-up adjustments, he did the same thing. It seemed as time went on the symptoms of cloudiness came back gradually, a little less each time. After several months he no longer had to return because the symptoms remained absent.

JOINT SOUNDS AND RESTRICTIONS

There can be noises in the joint, such as snapping, clicking, and popping sounds. These by themselves don't necessarily have to be treated, but often if they are getting worse or annoying everybody around a patient, they probably should be treated. The cause of these noises is usually some kind of damage to the engineering of the parts of the joints. If there are unusual strains on the ligaments and they can't perform properly, causing a recoiling of the disc all at once, this can create a "pop." There can also be abnormal shapes to the parts of the joint that can cause sounds. Each case should be evaluated with tomograms, a review of the patient's history, and mounted models in centric relation. It is generally accepted that noises shouldn't be treated unless pain is involved.

There are two other main causes of the noises. First is muscular restrictions. The muscles don't contract or relax smoothly, so they hold the disc a little too long as the jaw opens or closes. This type of problem responds well to correcting the bite. The most recent two cases I have corrected were of this type. One patient demonstrated a noticeable pop as he opened his mouth about a third of the way on the left side. The problem had started soon after he had retainers placed and had gradually gotten worse. After I finished the correction, which took only about an hour, the pop was gone.

The second other major cause is some type of anatomical dent or bump on the surface of the sliding parts of the joints. These will gradually get better but may never totally disappear. They took a long time to develop and will usually take a correspondingly long time to go away. They almost always start to improve immediately when the correct bite is restored.

Some jaw sounds are attributable to an arthritic problem. X-rays, MRIs, or CAT scans will usually show what's wrong. Muscle tenderness, pain, spasms, and cramps are important to note on the patient's list of problems. Although there is little correlation between the symptoms and the problem, we still need to have a thorough list to compare with post-treatment results.

RANGE OF MOTION LIMITATION

Range of motion can and should be part of the diagnosis of TMJ. It can tell us a lot about the health of the physical apparatus of the joint. If the jaw on opening deviates to the side instead of dropping straight down, that can tell us there is some kind of limitation in the TM joint on the same side. Some patients can't fully open their mouths. The muscles spasm, tense, cramp, or somehow tighten up so that they don't allow the full extension of the jaw. Very occasionally the bones themselves actually grow together and stop the movement of the jaw or severely limit it.

DISLOCATED JAW

And some folks actually can open too far and occasionally dislocate or lock their jaws apart. This condition usually succumbs to thumb pressure on the back teeth. The position of the condyle ahead of the eminence is usually obtained by a large yawn and the panic of tightening the muscles. Some relaxation and a little help from the dentist can fix it. Again, the severity of the problem is important to assess the need for treatment.

WHAT CAUSES TMJ?

When you close your teeth together, the TM joints automatically assume a specific posture. There isn't any way the bones and cartilage in the TM joints can change to accommodate a new posture or better posture unless you change the fit of the teeth.

THERE ARE ALWAYS TWO CAUSES TO A DISEASE. FIRST IS THE "PREDISPOSING" CAUSE AND SECOND THE "INCITING" CAUSE.

One of my favorite teachers was a professor of oral medicine at the University of Alabama, Emanuel Cheraskin, M.D., D.M.D. This wonderful, very articulate man published in the 1950s an article titled "The Arithmetic of Disease." In it he put forth the idea that there are always two causes to a disease. First is the "predisposing" cause and second the "inciting" cause. He stated "that it always takes two to tango." And he attached a value to each cause that allowed for a greater or lesser emphasis on any particular problem. For example, if you were chewing on an olive and suddenly found a pit when there wasn't supposed to be any and the instant strain on the TM joint was extreme, you could attach a 10 value to this event, 10 being the highest. This would be an "inciting" cause of TMJ. Then let's say that your mouth had a 3 millimeter slide with a 1 millimeter sideways deviation as the jaw moved forward from centric relation to centric occlusion and you had lived with it for fifty years—in other words, the worst malocclusion for quite a long time. Then you could attach a value of 10 to the "predisposing" cause. By now you recognize the patient has a major problem: 10 x 10 = 100, so according to our arithmetic, this patient would have a 100% chance of having TMJ. If the olive pit was a strawberry seed, and the patient had a perfect bite, the equation would be 1 x 1 instead of 10 x 10. These numbers are, of course, only approximate but provide an excellent way to conceptualize how TMJ is caused.

PREDISPOSING CAUSES

A predisposing cause of TMJ is some long-term slight strain or stress on the jaw joints. Some examples are: crooked or uneven teeth that don't fit correctly; worn, flat cusps on the teeth that disallow correct mastication and cause extra strain on the joints; and lack of proper occluding of the front teeth.

I have dealt with insurance companies that insist that the bite correction work I do isn't a covered benefit. They say to me: "The patient claims the auto accident produced the TMJ, and you are treating the patient with occlusal correction; doesn't that mean that the patient has a bad bite?" Then I have to reply, yes. Then they say they won't pay for that treatment because the bad bite pre-existed the auto accident. Most of the time I have to write a letter explaining that since I can't undo the auto accident straining the jaw joints, I have to fix the predisposing cause to "unload" the joints so they can heal quickly by themselves. I always like to use the example of the sprained ankle in high heels. Would the doctor do surgery on the ankle or take off the high heels? After all, the high heels didn't cause the sprain; the turned ankle caused it. Of course, the high heels may have increased the chance of a turned ankle. So does the bad bite increase the chances for TMJ, but it doesn't always cause it. The insurance people usually ask then whether the patient would have gotten the TMJ because of the bad bite. I have to say most likely not. The statistics and fifty-four years of experience show that most everyone has some type of a bad bite (malocclusion). Likewise, everyone doesn't have TMJ, but by some clinicians' estimates 20 percent of all people do. But I have to hedge a bit on this subject; I have seen patients come down with TMJ even though they never had any memorable insult to the joints. They simply had malocclusion long enough to wear down the resistance and bring it about. They had enough micro-traumas over a long enough period of time to start the TMJ.

Another form of "predisposing" causes is a weakness in the tissues themselves. There could be a number of minor anatomical factors that could possibly be involved, such as a loose ligament or too tight a ligament structure around the TM joints. These factors usually influence the healing time rather than the chances of healing.

TMJ can be cured by restoring the bite properly and taking away the unnecessary strains on the jaw joint. This concept is in conflict with current dental culture even though overwhelming evidence supports it. What is it that "they" don't understand about taking off the "high heels" for a sprained ankle?

INCITING CAUSES

There are many inciting causes of TMJ. A common one is whiplash as in a "rear-ended" automobile accident. The sudden blow from behind moves the body forward quickly, leaving the head behind. The neck must absorb the strain, which could be great or small depending on the severity of the blow. The strain probably stretches, possibly sprains, or even tears ligaments in the neck. Since the TM joint muscles and ligaments are either in common or very closely associated with the same muscle-ligament complex, there is shared damage. Now the controlling mechanisms of the chewing organ are damaged, namely the TM joints and their muscle-ligament complex. If a predisposing cause exists, say a malocclusion, then some level of TMJ will present itself. If the whiplash is severe, say 8–10 on a scale of 1–10, but the predisposing cause is only a 1 or 2, the TMJ may not present itself now but may manifest itself later. A person's

THERE ARE MANY INCITING CAUSES OF TMJ. A COMMON ONE IS WHIPLASH AS IN A "REAR-ENDED" AUTOMOBILE ACCIDENT.

nutritional intake, physical condition, and emotional health are part of the equation on the predisposing side. Any kind of injury to the jaws from falling, bicycling accidents, fighting, and biting accidents (pits, jerky, etc.) can trigger a TMJ episode. Even dentistry performed ignoring the bite can start TMJ. When implants are restored with bridgework or even single crowns, the common practice is to cement them too low. In other words, they don't support the proper bite. So the mouth may have only a few natural teeth to keep the proper vertical dimension. Frequently, the new crowns have little if any anatomy because they are probably not built into centric relation. The reason for this is the mouth was not corrected originally.

One of my most grievous complaints concerns the four bicuspid extraction practice of most all orthodontists. This practice is sold to the patient as the need for more room. "Too many teeth to put into those small jaws" they are told. But a very easy arch development with Crozat appliances removes the need for extraction and results in a superior facial appearance. This Crozat technique is not taught in orthodontic schools, and extractions frequently end up compromising most all the engineering requirements of organic occlusion.

CHAPTER 2

Today's Dental Occlusion

WHEN I GRADUATED from dental school, the term "TMJ" was never mentioned. We were taught anatomy of the head and neck very thoroughly, how to fill cavities, how to crown a tooth that had cavities too big to fill, how to clean teeth—but the temporomandibular joints were never mentioned. When we built a crown on a tooth, the fit of the edges was carefully checked. The fit of the crown to the tooth was regarded as very important, but the fit of the crown to the bite was not considered so important. The crown might be a little high, so we would grind it down, mostly because the patient would complain. The crown could be a little low so that it didn't even touch the opposite tooth. The patient wouldn't know that, and the instructors probably wouldn't know either.

Graduates today have learned many types of splint therapy, but few know what constitutes an ideal occlusion and how to change the bite to it. Let us assume for a moment that having an ideal occlusion would be the most likely cure to TMJ problems. That would mean that all dental schools would have to teach this perfect bite or occlusion, but sadly very few schools agree on what makes that perfect bite. Actually, most schools teach little about occlusion except how to build full upper and lower dentures. Mostly, the subject of occlusion is ignored. Postgraduate courses that teach full mouth reconstruction do begin to deal with it.

HISTORY AND EVOLUTION OF OCCLUSION

In the beginning there really was no concept; then we began to build false teeth (full dentures) and needed a scheme for arranging the teeth.

BALANCED OCCLUSION

This first effort was called "balanced occlusion." Briefly, the idea was that all the teeth rubbed as they traveled in all directions, left, right, and forward. The reason we believed in this was that we thought the dentures would stay in place better if they touched everywhere as they functioned. As you chewed food on one side of the mouth, the teeth touched on the other side, so it didn't tip and dislodge the dentures. Balanced occlusion seemed like a good idea, and some dentures are still based on this principle even today. In the 50s, however, balanced occlusion was found to be harmful to natural dentition.

CUSP-FOSSA OCCLUSION

This relationship is the most often seen in natural dentitions. Remember that the location of the teeth here doesn't say anything about the relationship to the TM joints, only how the upper teeth and lower fit against each other. This is not the ideal or final acceptable occlusion unless it coincides with the rearmost hinge position of the jaw (centric relation) and has immediate anterior disclusion. This topic will be explained fully in the next chapter on organic occlusion.

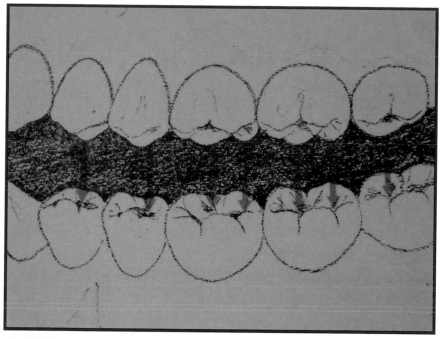

FIGURE 5: *Cusp-Fossa*

GROUP FUNCTION

This term refers to the worn dentition when the cuspid, premolars, and molars all fit together in a sideways movement of the mandible. It does not refer to how the teeth relate to the TM joints.

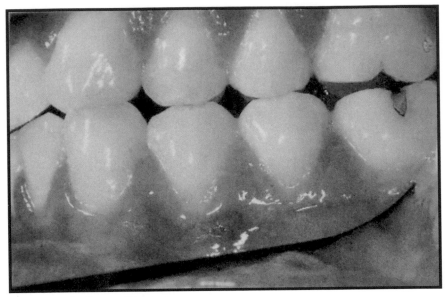

FIGURE 6: *Group Function*

MUTUALLY PROTECTED OCCLUSION

All these terms are used to describe some aspect of occlusion but don't fully explain it. It would be like describing how to drive a car by simple saying, "You put your foot on the gas pedal to make it go."

To understand this term, you have to divide the teeth into two parts: the front teeth, upper and lower, and all the back teeth, upper and lower. This begins to describe the "organic" nature of the dentition. When a person bites with the front teeth, he or she isn't using the back teeth. The muscles used are not used with much power. When the food bitten off is moved back to the chewing teeth, more power is used. Likewise, when the jaw is moved forward and opened a little where the front teeth meet, it is not in position to exert the most power. When the back teeth (chewing teeth) are in use, the jaw drops back where it has the most power and leverage. The closer the food is to the main one of the power muscles, called the masseter, the more power can be exerted. If you wanted to bite and chew the most resistant piece of tough steak, you would not try to do it with your front teeth.

"Mutually protected" also means that in the empty mouth, when the jaw slides forward or sideways, the front teeth separate the back teeth, thereby protecting them from lateral forces. Conversely, the posterior teeth protect the front teeth from heavy vertical forces because there's where we chew with the most power. The forward set protects the back set and vice versa.

ORGANIC OCCLUSION

This type of occlusion has been more recently discovered (about 1957) and embraces all the engineering principles necessary to relieve the TM joints from all stresses and allow the joints to heal. Therefore, we know it as the "ideal occlusion."

Unfortunately, it isn't taught in most dental schools and therefore isn't known by most dentists, much less by our physician friends.

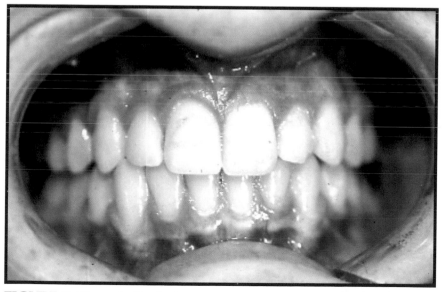

FIGURE 7: *Organic Occlusion*

It is the highest form of occlusion, the most natural, and the goal of every occlusal correction procedure. The engineering principles will be explained and compared to current practices in chapter 3.

When you look at this mouth (figure 7), you see a nice, straight, attractive set of teeth. Not only are they straight, but they also function properly. They exhibit organic occlusion. The jaw is seated properly in its fossae, and the teeth harmonize with that seated position of the jaw. (You can't see this.) Because of this harmony, there is no torque or pressure on the TM joints or the periodontal ligaments. The lower front teeth fit and touch the backs of the upper front teeth. Arches are properly developed, and the teeth stand upright in the bone. There is ample room for the tongue. Organic occlusion should be the ultimate goal of orthodontics, periodontics, and oral surgery.

> ORGANIC OCCLUSION SHOULD BE THE ULTIMATE GOAL OF ORTHODONTICS, PERIODONTICS, AND ORAL SURGERY.

IGNORANCE OR LACK OF TEACHING?

So why do you folks with TMJ have so much trouble finding help?

1. Occlusal correction is not taught in dental schools. The scientific literature predominately contradicts what I and most dentists believe. The literature says that the bite does not have any causal relation with TMJ.

2. Since occlusal correction is not taught in schools, splints and jaw surgery are frequently used. Both these procedures change the bite to a new wrong position and cost a lot of

money. Most of the time they fail to correct the bite and make things worse for the patient.

3. When a patient has an obvious bad bite, a dentist who believes as I do tries to correct the bite to help the patient. But because this procedure is very tricky, the attempt usually fails, leaving the patient worse and the dentist frustrated.

4. Because of the lack of knowledge or training of this dentist, the occlusal correction, when it fails, gives the procedure a bad name, which in turn reinforces the profession's objections to the procedure. It also reinforces the idea that the bite has nothing to do with TMJ.

5. The failure of this procedure can make dentists reluctant to attempt it, and this also helps to hide it from the public.

6. Like brain surgery in medicine, only very skilled dentists should be doing occlusal correction. They are called gnathologists.

7. This bite correction procedure is difficult and time consuming. There are disagreements among dentists as to which techniques remove the least amount of tooth structure. I say, "The less the better." The end product should always be the same: organic occlusion.

CHAPTER 3

Organic Occlusion

THIS CHAPTER EXPLAINS that there is a best way to fit teeth together rather than just any old way. The meeting of the lower jaw teeth against the upper jaw teeth is called occlusion. The prefix "organic" in this case means natural. If we did not say "organic," then it would not distinguish between just any meeting of the teeth and the highest and best type of occlusion.

I want to apologize to my readers for struggling to make a complicated subject simple. At the end of chapter 2, I outlined organic occlusion more for the public. In this chapter I've written more for the profession and in greater detail.

There are five requirements for organic occlusion:

1. Centric Jaw Relation
2. Immediate Anterior Disclusion
3. Cusp-Fossa Relationship
4. Stable, Even Bite
5. Cyclic Space

CENTRIC JAW RELATION

Centric jaw relation is the first and most important criterion for organic occlusion. We can describe this relationship as the "rearmost hinge position" of the mandible being in its socket. The jaw actually goes to this position when we swallow.

There are several ways to find this position. If you have been to a dentist who is making you a denture or other extensive dentistry, he or she may have pushed on your chin firmly and had you bite down on a piece of wax. The dentist was pushing your jaw back as far as it would go into "centric relation."

CENTRIC JAW RELATION IS THE FIRST AND MOST IMPORTANT CRITERION FOR ORGANIC OCCLUSION.

Another way to find "centric relation" is to jut your jaw forward as far as you can, like a bulldog, then bring it back with opposite muscles as far as you can without touching your teeth together. Then gently touch your teeth and observe how they fit. You at once realize they don't fit right and that isn't where you normally bite. Another way to find it is to put your head back as far as you can while looking at the ceiling or farther back and gently close your teeth together. With your head back the muscles under the chin are pulled taught, which forces the jaw back to the extreme limit. All these methods put the jaw in the rearmost hinge position, which by the way is the only repeatable position and the one we must use in finishing occlusal correction, orthodontics, periodontal treatment, jaw surgery, full mouth reconstruction, bridgework, implant replacements, partial dentures, full dentures, and in fact everything we do to replace missing or damaged teeth. We could probably do a root canal or a gum-line filling without being concerned about the bite.

IMMEDIATE ANTERIOR DISCLUSION

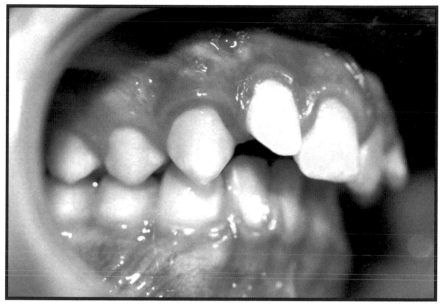

FIGURE 8: *Lack of immediate anterior disclusion*
"Overbite" and "overjet" combined. Lower anteriors are set too far back from the upper front teeth.

"Immediate" means that as soon as the jaw moves forward the backs of the upper front teeth cause the jaw to open and separate all the back teeth. "Anterior" means the front teeth. Normally, the front teeth touch when the back teeth are closed together. "Disclusion" means separation of teeth. As you can see in figure 8, the lower front teeth are about half an inch behind the backs of the upper front teeth, so as the jaw slides forward with teeth touching, the back teeth are hitting and crunching each other. The jaw does open but not with the front teeth. The jaw opens by the slopes of the back teeth, ramping at an angle against each other. They are contacting each other closer to the chewing muscles instead of further away like the front teeth. The increased forces push sideways instead of straight up and down on the posterior teeth. This interference also sets up detrimental forces on the TM joints and periodontal tissues and causes wear on the teeth. It sets up a teeter-totter effect on these back fulcrum teeth. This topic will be explored further in chapter 6, which will discuss the lever systems created by badly distorted bites.

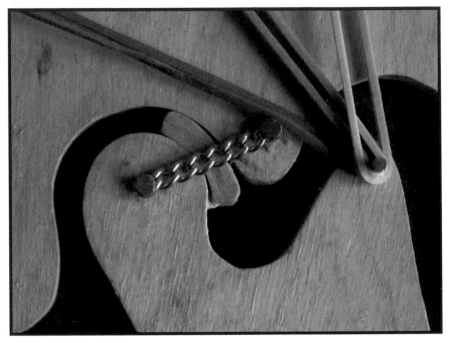

FIGURE 9: *Replica of TM joint.*
This is the back control of the chewing mechanism, with the condyle in the fossa. The gold chain represents the ligaments.

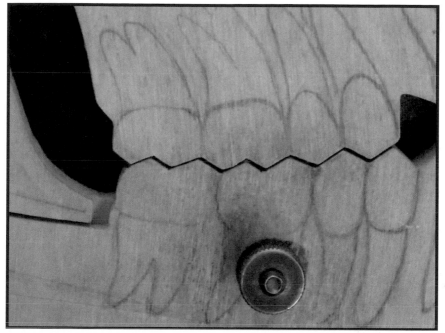

FIGURE 10: *Replica of the chewing teeth.*
The second and main part of the chewing mechanism.

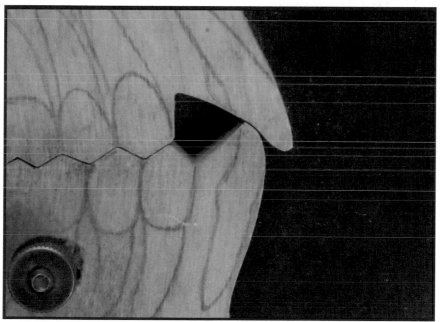

FIGURE 11: *Replica of the anterior teeth.*
The front control of the chewing mechanism. This model shows the anterior teeth touching. The slope of the back of the front tooth determines whether or not there will be immediate anterior disclusion.

But what if the slope is too flat or the upper is not touching the lower front tooth as in figure 8?

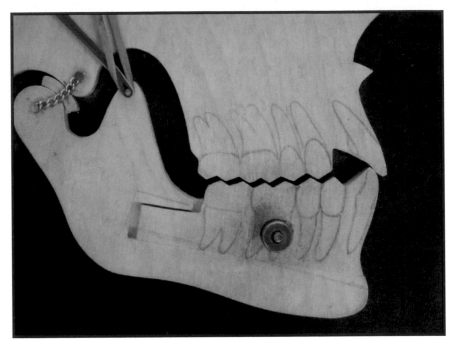

FIGURE 12: *Disclusion*
This shows the jaw sliding forward down the slope of the upper front teeth (front control) and all the teeth separating immediately. Notice that the chain in the joint is loose. The condyle is sliding down the slope of the eminence and is allowing the teeth to separate.

So we have the TM joint with the eminence and the backs of the anterior teeth as the two control systems, one in front and one in back to separate the chewing teeth. If the front teeth don't separate, then the chewing teeth have to do that, causing wear and lateral forces on those teeth. The posterior teeth are designed to resist vertical forces more than lateral ones. That is why they all have shorter roots. The upper front teeth all have longer roots and therefore are designed to resist lateral forces because they are farther away from the powerful chewing muscles and their resistance for displacement is greater. So the design of immediate anterior disclusion causes the oral chewing organ to function properly, protecting the posterior teeth from lateral forces. This is also called mutually protected occlusion, discussed in the last chapter. Having the TM joint in the rearmost hinge position and the front teeth touching while all the posterior chewing teeth are together is the ideal or organic bite.

HAVING THE TM JOINT IN THE REARMOST HINGE POSITION AND THE FRONT TEETH TOUCHING WHILE ALL THE POSTERIOR CHEWING TEETH ARE TOGETHER IS THE IDEAL OR ORGANIC BITE.

CUSP-FOSSA RELATIONSHIP

This term refers mainly to the fit of the posterior teeth. Cusps are the points on the tops of the posterior teeth. Fossae are the depressions or valleys on the tops of the back teeth in which the cusps fit. (See figures 13 and 14.) The cusps of the upper fit into the fossae of the lower in a precise way. (See figure 15.) They have ridges and grooves that harmonize with the chewing motions of the jaw and properly masticate the food. They don't rub together unless the number one and two requirements are missing. They do come close but only touch when in the final center rearmost position and the mouth is empty.

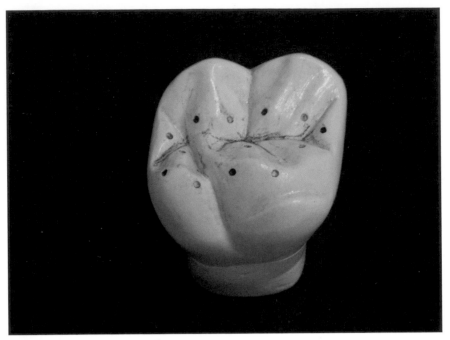

FIGURE 13: *Upper molar*

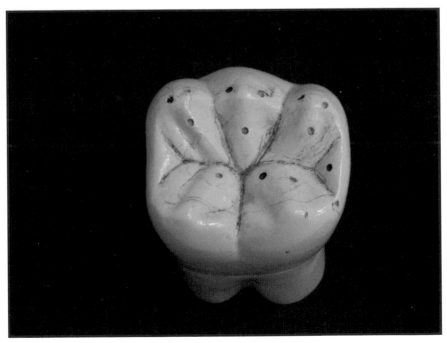

FIGURE 14: *Lower molar*

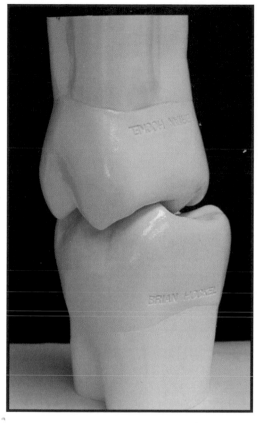

FIGURE 15: *Upper and lower molars occluded together* This relationship is stable and connected by the tripod points surrounding each cusp, indicated by the red and black dots in figures 13 and 14. Models courtesy of Brian Hockel, DDS.

When the jaws move forward or sideways from "centric relation," the cusps lift off from the contacting position like an airplane taking off from the landing runway. The individual teeth have a specific way of fitting together. When the teeth have all grown in to their best fit, the jaw has a specific location also. If the jaw can't find a specific location, then in an effort to find one, a person may start to grind the teeth (i.e., bruxing).

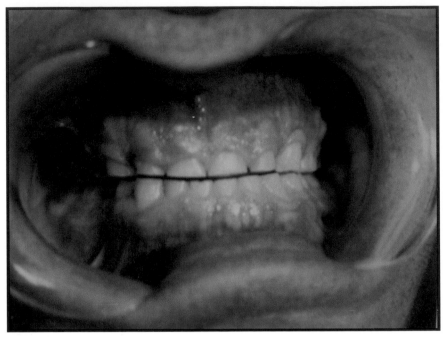

FIGURE 16: *Severe bruxism*
This person is twenty-nine years old. He couldn't remember when he started to grind.

When the jaw can't find a definite location to bite, there is a subconscious urge to grind or clench, to try to find a stable position. After many reconstruction, occlusal correction, and orthodontic cases I have completed, the patients tell me they don't have that tendency to grind anymore. That change of feeling happened immediately when the proper organic occlusion was installed.

WHEN THE JAW CAN'T FIND A DEFINITE
LOCATION TO BITE, THERE IS A SUBCONSCIOUS
URGE TO GRIND OR CLENCH, TO TRY TO FIND
A STABLE POSITION.

When the cusps and fossae are worn flat or nearly so, the bite becomes a skating rink and increases the tendency to brux. Flat teeth don't work. Flat teeth can mash the food to some degree, but normal chewing is not possible. Remember that if requirements one and two are missing, the posterior teeth will wear, increasing the risk for periodontal disease and the torque on the TM joints.

The tops of the teeth have a secret set of messages that dentistry has mostly ignored. The ridge and groove direction and the cusp height and fossa depth have been locked out of mainstream dentistry, which doesn't want to consider that there are engineering principles that confirm all these principles that "gnathology" embraces.

The steepness or flatness of the cusps is all in harmony with the shape of the TM joints. When you consider the arcing circles of the lower jaw as it chews, you realize that there have to be controls in the TM joints that harmonize with the shapes of the tops of the teeth. More specifically, there are slopes in the TM joints and the anatomy of the backs of the upper front teeth. They dictate the direction of travel of the lower jaw. The front teeth influence the front part of the jaw, and the slopes in the TM joints influence the back part. The amount of influence varies with the distance forward or backward.

THE TOPS OF THE TEETH HAVE A SECRET SET OF MESSAGES THAT DENTISTRY HAS MOSTLY IGNORED.

Let's say that the travel of the jaw is relatively flat due to the formation in the TM joints. Then, if a dentist tried to replace missing teeth with implants or bridgework with steep, pointed cusps, the cusps probably would not separate when the patient would chew. The lifting controls of the TM joints wouldn't fit with the steep interlocking cusps and fossae. Interferences are induced and torque against the other parts of the oral mechanism. Many dental offices lacking knowledge of organic occlusion get away with the mistakes because of the human capacity to adapt and get over most anything. But shouldn't dentistry have the responsibility to at least know when to stop guessing? This third requirement is necessary to harmonize with the other requirements of organic occlusion.

STABLE, EVEN BITE

"Stable" means that when the teeth touch together, there is no slippage. A three-legged stool is stable on any level surface. The teeth should meet vertically without any shift or slide when each opponent set meets with a tripod contact. (See figures 13, 14, and 15.) This stability depends on the jaw being in the centric related position (the first requirement).

"Stable" also means there is no orthodontic movement or drifting. Think about teeth to the rear of an extracted tooth space. There is no tooth in front of these teeth to lean against. There is a normal natural forward movement or drifting tendency that is built into the system to keep the contacts of the teeth together. If there is an extraction without replacement, then there is a lack of stability. When four good teeth are extracted for orthodontic correction, usually the arch is contracted by tipping teeth toward the tongue. Then the vertical alignment of opposing teeth is lost, and the vertical force of the bite can tip the teeth farther in toward the tongue.

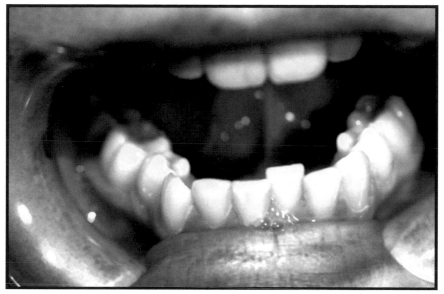

FIGURE 17: *Lower arch contracted*
A lower arch contracted with two lower bicuspids extracted and the spaces closed by tipping the teeth inward. Tongue space is diminished.

"Even" means the teeth all meet at the same time. There is no discrepancy from one side of the bite to the other. When teeth are missing, there can be drifting and intrusion of one side of the mouth to the other. Then there can be a difference of height between the two sides.

If one tooth hits before another, it can: 1) damage the tooth and cause its loss; 2) create a teeter-totter effect, which causes strain on the TM joints; 3) put too much pressure on the root and cause the gum to recede or periodontal problems. It just makes good sense to have all the teeth hit at the same time. What can and does happen when we perform some kind of restorative dentistry is some teeth can be built up too high. My guess is that virtually everyone has had a high filling placed and had to return the next day to their dentist to have it ground down slightly. The reason this happens is the dentist can't detect the high spots without the patient's help. So when the patient's pressure-sensitive mechanism isn't working because of a local anesthetic, the high spot doesn't show up in the dental chair. The amount of highness may well have been less than 10 microns. The patient can feel discrepancies that small, but the dentist isn't capable of measuring them.

CYCLIC SPACE

Cyclic space refers to the space inside the mouth. It could also be referred to as the volume inside the mouth. There are several parts to this requirement. First, the volume of the mouth should be large enough for a fully developed tongue. Often, with a four bicuspid orthodontic extraction case the arch can be diminished enough to encroach on the tongue space.

MUSCLES WILL ALWAYS WIN AGAINST BONE.

Second, it refers to the height of space between the upper and lower jaws, which is called "vertical dimension." This space is very difficult to determine when fabricating false teeth (full dentures). There is no exact way to measure it without teeth in both arches that meet. The way dentists try to measure it is with verbal tricks like saying "mmm" and measuring with marks on the upper lip and chin. We call it instinct and educated guesses. We depend on the muscles of the jaws to tell us this dimension.

The length of the chewing muscles does not change, and when the vertical dimension is measured with "mmm," the patient should be close to the centric occlusion position. There should be about 3–5 mm of closure, which is called the "freeway space." This space should not be violated with splints or night guards. The muscles need this space to rest, and the muscles will always win against bone.

Third, there are obstacles to the normal chewing cycle, such as misaligned teeth that cause bumps to the smooth travel of the teeth from side to side. Cross bites of front teeth are examples of this. Teeth that are crowded out of the arch toward the tongue can also be obstacles.

So these five requirements constitute organic occlusion. They are interdependent. We must not leave even one out when complete treatment is expected, but the first two are the most important.

Dr. Gus Swab tells us, "Organic Occlusion is the arrangement of teeth that happily fits into the oral organ without violating group uses of teeth, length of chewing muscles, interocclusal space, rest position, and condylar controls. As dentists we must be aware of the signs, symptoms and degrees of 'happiness' of the oral organ."

Toothaches are easy; periodontal disease a little more difficult; but TMJ is probably the most trying problem in our work. TMJ can be cured but not as soon as we would like. Toothaches can be dealt with within hours or even minutes. Periodontal disease requires a long-term consistent, repetitious, and diligent effort. TMJ is like that also. Organic occlusion must be installed, then maintained very accurately for a period of time. The longer the malocclusion exists, the longer the healing time.

ORGANIC OCCLUSION MUST BE INSTALLED, THEN MAINTAINED VERY ACCURATELY FOR A PERIOD OF TIME. THE LONGER THE MALOCCLUSION EXISTS, THE LONGER THE HEALING TIME.

CHAPTER 4

Occlusion Culture

THERE SEEMS TO BE a major disagreement involving the concept of jaw location in the jaw socket or TM joint. There are several possibilities to consider. As we described in the chapter on anatomy, the part of the jaw bone that fits into the socket is called the condyle. The socket is part of the temporal bone just ahead of the ear opening.

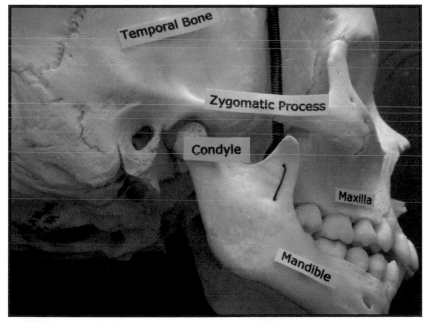

FIGURE 18: *Skull with labels on the bones*

The mandible is held in place by ligaments (figure 3) that keep it from impinging on the very thin bone separating the TM joint from the ear. The ligaments are very strong in order to prevent the mandible from traveling rearward as when a knockout blow to the chin is delivered during a prize fight.

This replica of the skull in figure 19 shows the condyle connected to the bone in front with a small gold chain, which duplicates the activity of the ligaments. Notice how as the jaw moves rearward the condyle rotates upward and forward around the pin at the front end of the gold chain. The elastics represent the temporalis muscle. The posterior fibers of that muscle, represented by the blue elastic, pull the mandible rearward. The other two elastics pull upward and more forward, all part of the temporalis muscle shown in figure 20.

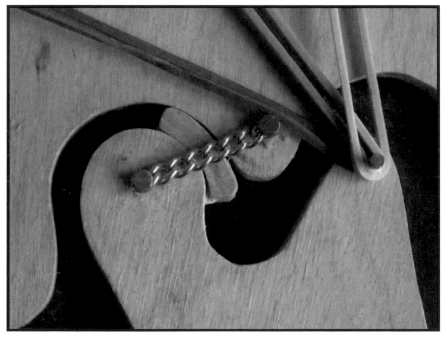

FIGURE 19: *Replica of the TM joint*

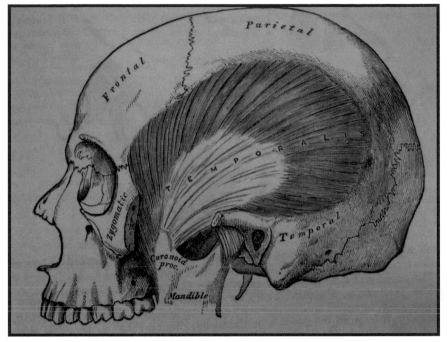

FIGURE 20: *The temporalis muscle*

ARGUMENT

So this argument is whether it matters where the condyle is located when the teeth are completely shut. Should the condyle be completely rearward, or can it be forward of the rearmost position? The replica shown in figure 9 shows the gold chain taut, meaning the jaw is in the rearmost position. In this replica the posterior fibers of the temporalis muscle are pulling the jaw into that rearmost position (CR).

Mainstream dentistry recognizes that the average patient walks into an office with the jaw location, when he or she bites down, not in the rearmost position. So when the average patient is not in centric relation, we find it very easy to ignore what is best and just do normal dentistry.

TODAY'S DENTISTRY

Most simple dentistry, such as fillings, root canals, and pro-phylaxis, doesn't require *changing the bite*. As I have stated before, TMJ treatment *does* require changing the bite to organic occlusion. Since organic occlusion (see chapter 3) is the latest concept of occlusion, most dentists either haven't been trained to use it, don't want to use it, or are oblivious to it. The preponderance of dental literature is equally guilty.

> SINCE ORGANIC OCCLUSION IS THE LATEST CONCEPT OF OCCLUSION, MOST DENTISTS EITHER HAVEN'T BEEN TRAINED TO USE IT, DON'T WANT TO USE IT, OR ARE OBLIVIOUS TO IT.

PART OF THE PROBLEM

Most dental offices have multiple operating rooms because dentists believe that multiple rooms are more time efficient. The downside to that is they need more space and more personnel to run their offices. In my office I also found multiple operating rooms discouraged conversation and rapport, and they raised the cost of my operating. When I became a gnathologist and was schooled in what the bite was supposed to be and how to get it there, I had to sell my practice and switch from five operatories to one chair with a large laboratory in order to do my own lab work. My stress level went down, and my quality of service went up. My overhead went from about 80 percent of finances down to about 20 percent. Now I had time to talk to my patients and explain the need to change the bite to the rearmost posture (organic occlusion). Suddenly, there occurred a change in my practice, resulting in the need for a major training sabbatical.

RELUCTANCE TO CHANGE

Over the years I have witnessed that there seems to be, in any profession, a terrible resistance to change. Looking at the medical profession in the cancer treatment area, for example, the author of an article in one of the last alternative medicine newsletters I receive tells of a celebration of thirty years of curing cancer. It took place in Houston, Texas, at Stanislaw Burzynski's clinic. The author saw and talked with hundreds of post-terminal patients who were reveling in the joy of being alive. The discovery of novel peptides in the blood that were absent in cancer patients challenged this Polish researcher to synthesize the peptides and treat patients, thereby shrinking and eliminating tumors. I asked myself why this event wasn't instant headline news in all the media? Could it be a disbelief of the validity of the treatment or just a reluctance to change, similar to the reluctance of dentists to make use of occlusal correction?

ANOTHER PART OF THE PROBLEM—SPLINTS

A problem with TMJ treatment is the difficulty with changing the bite. But mainstream dentistry has solved that by inventing the bite "splint." It is a time saver for the average office, which tries to change the existing incorrect or painful bite to a new incorrect bite. The patient can be treated by the usual quick impressions of the teeth, which are poured with plaster and then sent to a lab that fabricates the splint. When the patient returns, the splint may be placed in the mouth, possibly by someone on the staff. The doctor may adjust and explain the care and use of the splint. Much more is said about splints in chapter 5.

THE REFERRAL SYSTEM

When a patient visits his or her dentist for a normal check-up, nothing is mentioned about the bite, whether it is off or just "okay." The subject of gum tissue health is almost always discussed. Pocket depth measurements are taken and recorded on a chart. Patients are schooled in how to brush and use certain tooth medications. X-rays are taken and defects charted.

Then, when a TMJ "inciting cause" takes place, the patient seeks the advice of his or her dentist for the TMJ pain, which necessitates that the dentist bring a whole new area of expertise to bear. Maybe the dentist wasn't schooled for it. So, often the patient is referred to a professional who is thought to be trained for TMJ. Possibly this dentist is an oral surgeon, who is pleased to receive the referral and is obligated to treat the TMJ. Is this oral surgeon trained to treat TMJ, though? He or she is probably not. His or her training has probably been in surgery and perhaps splints. Few general dentists or oral surgeons are trained to do full mouth bite correction. What if the surgeon knew that the bite was off? He or she would refer the patient to a gnathologist, who is another general dentist. Then probably the original referring dentist wouldn't send the surgeon any more patients. So the oral surgeon is likely to try to go ahead and treat the patient with splints or possibly open TM joint surgery. The dentist and the surgeon keep their patients, but the patients receive poor treatment. I believe that the lack of training of the average dentist causes this problem.

FEW DENTISTS REALLY REALIZE THAT THE NATURAL TEETH NEED THE SAME MECHANICS AND ENGINEERING AS FALSE TEETH NEED.

FULL DENTURES
(FALSE TEETH–PLATES)

Few dentists really realize that the natural teeth need the same mechanics and engineering as false teeth need. General dentists were taught in dental school how to make dentures. Unfortunately, the dental laboratories usually inherit the job after the dentist graduated.

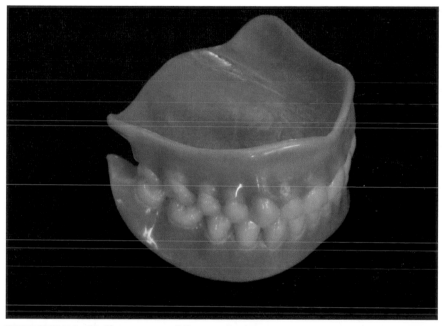

FIGURE 21: *Full upper and lower dentures*

The fact that full dentures only work in centric relation further verifies the use of the rearmost posture of the mandible. One of the simple and most neglected engineering principles is: If it is already there, it can't move any further back. This is part of the engineering principles of organic occlusion discussed in detail in chapter 3.

PERIODONTAL DISEASE

When the jaw is rearmost, the closure is an exact location, and when we correct the teeth to coincide with that location, the teeth are comfortable and do not interfere with each other. There is no violence in the mouth. Interference results when there is a "hit and slide" bite. When the jaw is not in the centric relation (rearmost) and the teeth close together, they strike each other at an angle.

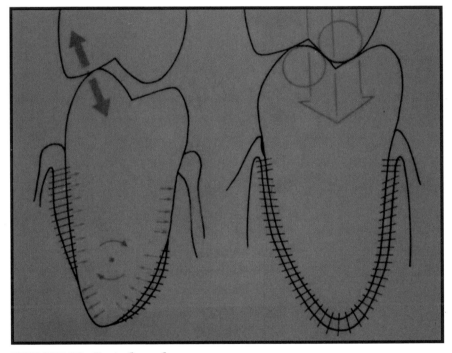

FIGURE 22: *Periodontal cause*

This problem can contribute to *periodontal disease*. Figure 22 shows two teeth: One hits at an angle to push the tooth out of its socket whereas the other hits with its correct tripod contact. Since the average dentist is taught to chart the pocket depth at checkup time, why not have mounted study models in centric relation to show the evidence of the chief cause of periodontal disease? Normally during a checkup a dentist is trying to find and correct all deficiencies, whether tooth or gum. That means the examination has left out or ignored the need for charting the bite. The occlusion of a patient's teeth has to be the most important item for the diagnosis of TM joint health, periodontal health, and wearing or grinding the teeth. In gnathology, occlusion is the first requirement to maintain good longevity for the mouth, not the last. Occlusion should come first in a routine dental checkup, not last or be forgotten altogether. For me, the most spectacular reason for organic occlusion is that *it works*. It satisfies all the requisites of a peaceful, comfortable, and healthy mouth and surrounding structures.

IN GNATHOLOGY, OCCLUSION IS THE FIRST
REQUIREMENT TO MAINTAIN GOOD LONGEVITY
FOR THE MOUTH, NOT THE LAST.

CHAPTER 5

TMJ Treatment by Mainstream Dentists

YOU CALL YOUR dentist for an appointment, and the well-spoken receptionist you have known for many years makes you one for next Tuesday at 9:30 A.M. You get there about 9:20, are greeted, and are told the doctor is running a little late. So you read the most recent *People* magazine till you are told at about 9:45 that the doctor is behind because of extra procedures he or she had to do. No problem, because you planned on a little extra time here.

But today's visit is different than just cleaning and X-rays. Today you woke with a sore jaw problem and a headache. What am I dealing with here? you ask yourself. Maybe it is cancer? Finally, the doctor takes you in and begins the questioning. Did it just start today? How bad on a scale of 1–10, 10 being the worst? X-rays are taken and compared with those taken maybe a year and a half ago. Nothing shows up on the new X-rays. Your dentist taps on the tops of the teeth to see whether any of them are questionable to percussion. That might be a clue to an abscess. Finally, the dentist believes the problem lies with the TM joint. After taking impressions of the teeth, the dentist advises you that he or she is making you a splint to support your bite and relieve your headaches.

SPLINTS

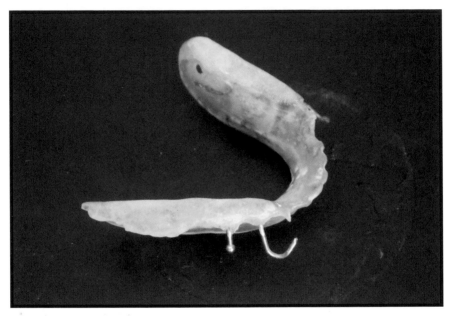

FIGURE 23: *A lower splint*

For large clinics and most "mainstream" dentists splints are the choice of treatment. Splints can provide immediate relief and hope for the patient, but the reason for the relief is really a testimony as to what is wrong—the habitual bite or the fit of the natural teeth is wrong. A splint, therefore, is, at best, a temporary form of treatment but can produce immediate relief from the pain. There are many forms of splints, but unfortunately they all open the bite. So they should be used only temporarily. Often the dentist prescribes a splint but doesn't explain what should come after this temporary treatment—namely, "occlusal correction."

SPLINTS CAN PROVIDE IMMEDIATE RELIEF AND
HOPE FOR THE PATIENT, BUT THE REASON FOR
THE RELIEF IS REALLY A TESTIMONY AS TO WHAT
IS WRONG—THE HABITUAL BITE OR THE FIT OF
THE NATURAL TEETH IS WRONG.

If you place foreign material like a splint between the teeth (opening the bite), nature causes the muscles to squeeze the bite and force an orthodontic intrusion of the teeth. The teeth will actually sink into the bone. The muscles need space to rest, and when you fill this space with teeth, something has to give. When the teeth first grow into the mouth, they continue to grow in until they touch each other. Then they stop erupting or growing in. If they grow in too far, the chewing muscles soon push them down to the right place. There is a dynamic equilibrium between the eruption of the teeth and the growth of the chewing muscles.

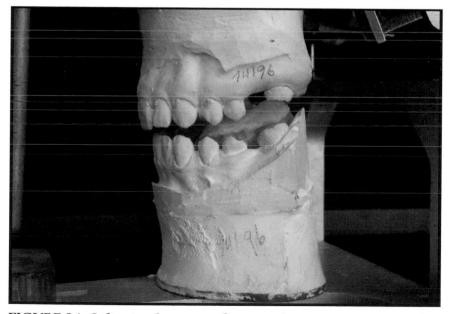

FIGURE 24: *Splint in place worn for several years*

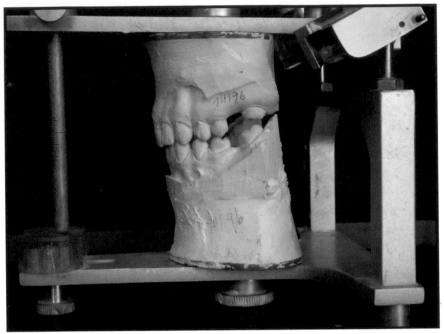

FIGURE 25: *Splint taken out and the mouth closed down*
Notice how the front teeth touch and the rear teeth are three-eighths of an inch apart.

So if you artificially lengthen the teeth (with a splint), the muscles push the teeth down to the right level. You can't fool the muscles. The same is true with the tongue and lips. They control the location of teeth in between themselves. If the tongue is too big, the teeth tip outwardly and usually have spaces between them. If the lips are too strong and tight, the teeth lean inwardly and usually overlap and are crooked. These are the natural orthodontic controls.

I have seen photos of teeth that have intruded even more until the tops of the teeth were level with the gums. The reason for this is simple. As I have said before, if there is a war between muscle and bone, muscle always wins.

Here is an example I read about years ago: A fellow who wanted to be taller went to a surgeon, who made steep diagonal incisions in the long bones of the leg to lengthen the bones. After healing, the patient was an inch taller. Unfortunately, a year later he was back to the same height. He forgot that the muscles remained the same length. Bone conforms to the muscle. In the case of splints, if you open the bite with a splint, eventually something has to change to satisfy the length of the chewing muscles. We call this "vertical orthodontics."

You should know that when a splint is the treatment, there needs to be a correction done in some way to get rid of the splint. When splints are worn, the normal bite gets worse and harder to correct. The patients are literally "married" to them. Teeth intrude, and then when proper treatment is commenced, the teeth seem to erupt at different rates of speed. This slows proper treatment and healing. If the splint is only covering the back teeth, then only the back teeth will intrude. If the splint covers only the front teeth, then only the front teeth will intrude. If the splint covers all the teeth, all the teeth intrude. The thicker the splint, the faster the intrusion takes place. The more the splint is worn, the faster the intrusion takes place.

Usually, splints are made out of plastic. They provide a quick and easy way to change the bite temporarily, but the bite on the splint is only approximate. The plastic is slightly soft and not capable of being carved into the proper anatomy or of holding the shape of that anatomy. So the bite can never be made right on plastic. Even if you took the trouble to create the correct and accurate anatomy, it wouldn't last but a few weeks, and then it would be worn out again.

Sometimes a splint needs to be made to relieve the pain enough to perform a proper diagnosis. Occasionally, I have made a splint out of gold to shim one area of the bite to make it level with the other side. This is a much thinner piece with better anatomy, causing less intrusion.

Splints are the primary treatment for TMJ from the "main-stream" dentists. It is not so much that splints are a bad treatment as it is that they are sold to the public as almost the only form of treatment.

ORTHODONTICS

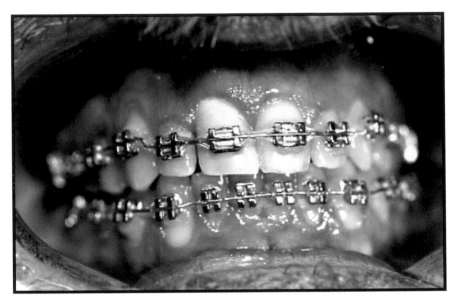

FIGURE 26: *Braces*

Orthodontics, moving the teeth, will immediately help most TMJ sufferers. The minute you start moving the teeth, you have changed the old bite. The adverse forces on the TM joints have changed. Anything that changes the wrong habitual bite will provide temporary relief. In orthodontia, you continually change the bite until you finish into retainers, and then as the retainers hold the teeth into the finished position, the TMJ pain can come thundering back if the bite isn't corrected to the organic position.

ORTHODONTICS IS AN EXCELLENT TREATMENT FOR TMJ AS LONG AS THE FINISHED CASE EMBRACES ORGANIC OCCLUSION.

Another reason the orthodontic treatment stops the TMJ pain is that the teeth as they start to move get spongy in their sockets. They have a little give to them, a shock-absorbing quality. This in and of itself can relieve TMJ. I always advise my patients while they are under treatment that the pains can come and go and sometimes even get worse than they were to start with. Unfortunately, I have seen all too many "finished" orthodontic cases that didn't have organic occlusion and required splints maybe forever. So orthodontics is an excellent treatment for TMJ as long as the finished case embraces organic occlusion.

TM JOINT SURGERY

With the great improvement of diagnostic techniques for TMJ, it has become easier to see and record what defects are actually present in the TM joint itself. Improved diagnostic techniques create a great temptation to try to fix TMJ by surgical intervention. I strongly recommend you don't take this route. When dentists first realized that this disease of the TM joint caused anatomical changes in the joint, X-rays were taken. These first X-rays were called "transcranials." Then, improved techniques were introduced, which were necessary because with transcranials the image was a profile of the condyle and left out valuable information hidden behind the silhouette. Now we have excellent images (tomograms) that are slices through the bone and tissues showing the joint completely.

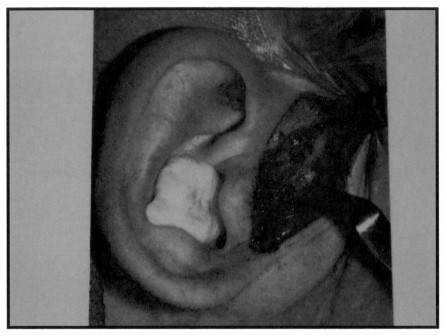

FIGURE 27: *A surgically exposed TM joint*

IMPROVED DIAGNOSTIC TECHNIQUES CREATE
A GREAT TEMPTATION TO TRY TO FIX TMJ BY
SURGICAL INTERVENTION. I STRONGLY
RECOMMEND YOU DON'T TAKE THIS ROUTE..

ARTHROSCOPY

The first and most non-invasive efforts were arthroscopy in nature. The interior of the two joint spaces could be observed and irrigated, and very limited surgery was performed. This technique has had some beneficial results that couldn't be achieved in other ways. Open joint surgery seldom is indicated but is often abused in treatment of TMJ. It has been said by many that open TM joint surgery is a very last resort. I personally have seen many open TM joint surgeries used when the incorrect bite was totally ignored. The open surgery of the TM joint should be prevented at all costs. When bite correction is over 90 percent successful and over 90 percent ignored by the surgeons, something is radically wrong.

JAW REDUCTION SURGERY

In TMJ work, orthodontia becomes necessary when the teeth are so far from their proper positions that occlusal correction cannot be utilized. Taking this a step farther, when the jaws are too far from their normal position to be corrected with orthodontics, then jaw surgery is necessary. So when a TMJ case is analyzed for treatment, the normal tooth and jaw position is determined and compared to what is presented for treatment. A set of mounted study models show these important relationships. Then, if the teeth are in a reasonably normal position and the jaws are also, occlusal correction is utilized to calibrate the bite into harmony with the TM joints. If the jaws are normally configured but the teeth don't allow the occlusal correction to work, then orthodontics is the choice. When the jaws are too far out of normal alignment for orthodontics to work, then jaw surgery is necessary. Then orthodontics is used to ready the teeth for surgery, then to finalize, after surgery, occlusal correction to finish to the accuracy necessary to achieve organic occlusion.

The need for jaw surgery is not always clear. My practice in the past has been to attempt to move the teeth into their normal relationships first; then, if this just doesn't get the relationships close enough to create organic occlusion, surgery is needed. It suddenly becomes clear what needs to be done in these questionable cases when they are diagnosed on an articulator and the plaster teeth are cut off the bases and set in wax to organic occlusion. This procedure is called a "positioner set up" and is mostly utilized to make positioners out of hard elastic plastic to be worn in the mouth a few months in order to finalize orthodontic cases. This device looks much like a sports mouth guard that is worn to protect the teeth during athletic events. There are orthodontic uses of this procedure called "Invisiline," which utilizes a series of positioners, each one formed a little closer to straight teeth. This technique has helped a limited number of types of malocclusion cases but can save the patient from fixed appliances.

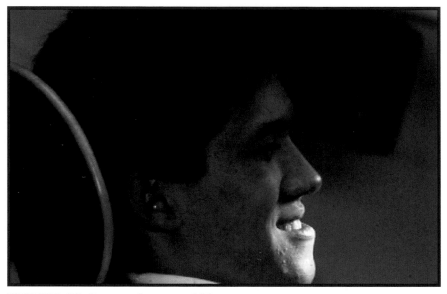

FIGURE 28: *Prognathic mandible*

Occasionally, jaw surgery is necessary to reduce the size of one of the jaws (usually the mandible), as in figure 28, so as to bring the teeth together properly. Sometimes it is necessary to move the upper jaw forward of its position to increase its size and to make the teeth fit. Sometimes it's also necessary to move both upper and lower jaws to make the teeth meet properly. Bear in mind that this surgery takes place in the "body" of the mandible, not in the TM joint. I have found jaw surgery necessary many times in my practice but rarely, practically never, TM joint surgery.

MISCELLANEOUS THERAPIES

Physical therapy can help rehabilitate TMJ cases, along with hypnosis, biofeedback, meditation, and muscle stimulation with TENS units. I mention these just to round out the list of techniques used by "mainstream" dentists and oral surgeons. Just think about all these techniques listed above: splints, orthodontics, TMJ surgery. Splints don't produce organic occlusion. Orthodontics can produce it, if the orthodontist knows organic occlusion. TM joint surgery doesn't change the bite. Physical therapy, chiropractics, biofeedback, meditation, and TENS stimulation don't change the bite. Who, I ask, can fix the bite? Burt Reynolds can tell you.

CHAPTER 6

Treatment by Gnathology

MRS. JONES IS IN terrible pain with her jaw joints. She has just now bitten on an olive pit that wasn't supposed to be there. She immediately calls her dentist for help. Dr. Smith answers the phone and asks her to come in immediately. Mrs. Jones notices that he has only one chair, instead of five or so, and a large laboratory. He looks at her teeth and checks her X-rays. She can't open and close very well but manages to sit through the examination. Muscles are palpated, range of motion recorded, teeth are checked, and history taken. Discussion centers on the cause and future treatment.

THE COTTON-BALL TREATMENT

For now the cotton-ball treatment is recommended until the pain subsides in this TMJ case. Splints are discussed for temporary relief but should not be used for longer than six weeks or so. The cotton-ball treatment is selected until models are taken and mounted to find the "predisposing" cause of the TMJ pain. A small ball of cotton the size of a pencil eraser is placed in the mouth between the back teeth, so that when the person bites down, he or she will feel the cotton and not clench together. It doesn't matter on which side the cotton is placed. It prevents the misaligned teeth from touching and prevents the adverse pressure on the TM joints. The person still has to eat, so he or she is instructed to eat just very soft foods or soup till the bite is corrected. The cotton ball is used immediately after eating and all the rest of the time. Patients can easily keep it in at night. If swallowed, there is no problem. The cotton is always moist so it isn't inhaled. This form of treatment is not only inexpensive but also very effective. What we desire here is to take the pressure off the "sprained ankle" effect of the TMJ.

SLEEPING INSTRUCTIONS

Along with the cotton ball in the mouth, the patient is instructed to sleep on his or her back or side. When placing the pillow, the person should move his or her jaw back and forth to make sure there is no pressure on the lower jaw at all. This kind of extra pressure on the jaw joint while sleeping could be detrimental to the healing process.

The patient is reappointed and let go with instructions to call if there is any problem. When she returns, models are taken (two sets) and mounted.

Centrically related wax bites and a face bow are taken to mount the models on a Whipmix articulator.

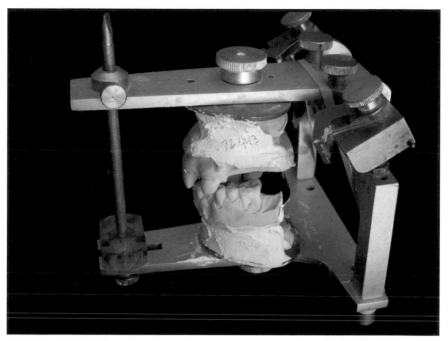

FIGURE 29: *Whipmix articulator with mounted models*

When the patient returns, the models are shown as before and after correction.

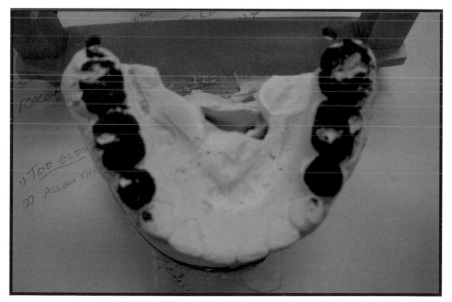

FIGURE 30: *Red poster paint on mounted models*

Red poster paint is put on the tops of the posterior teeth, and then cuts are made according to the interferences to correct the bite. The models are shown to the patient and explanations made about how very small cuts on the tops of the teeth are done.

These corrected models are then retained, along with the original maloccluded models as part of the patient's permanent record. These corrected models are also used as a guide to make the same cuts in the mouth when the occlusal correction procedure is performed on the patient. This rarely used procedure is the main teaching of gnathology.

Gnathos is a Greek word meaning "jaws," and *-ology* indicates the science thereof—thus, "gnathology." Harvey Stallard, DDS, one of the first to discover the science and engineering principles of the oral organ, gave us this name. When you consider that the jaw rotates around something and you look at the anatomy of the TM joint, you begin to realize that there are engineering principles involved. Forces at certain angles applied to the teeth and jaws begin to cause us to realize that nature set up certain rules of engagement. Class 1, class 2, and class 3 lever systems are involved when we consider these forces.

GNATHOS IS A GREEK WORD MEANING "JAWS," AND *-OLOGY* INDICATES THE SCIENCE THEREOF— THUS, "GNATHOLOGY."

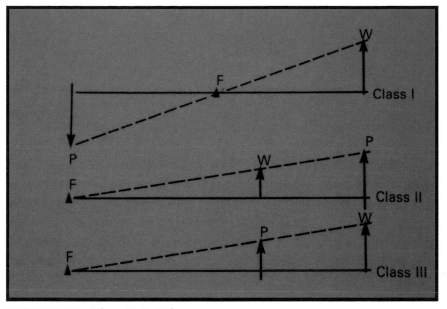

FIGURE 31: *Class 1, 2, 3 levers*

When dentistry began in the barbershop with a bottle of whiskey and a pair of forceps, little attention was paid to cavities that caused toothaches, much less to the TM joints. We have come a long way, but most dentists are still practicing "one-tooth dentistry." The dental schools rarely teach gnathology to the undergraduate. Postgraduate courses are where most dentists learn the complexities of orthodontics, periodontics, pedodontics, endodontics, and oral surgery. Some schools teach some gnathology in their advanced prosthodontics courses. Not all of this teaching is pure gnathology. Most of the true gnathologists did not receive any advanced training but were only practicing general dentists. I mention this only to explain the evolution of gnathology. It came from individuals who grasped these missing engineering principles that mainstream teachers were neglecting. There were problems that our dental schools had no answers for. This led to the development of the first "articulators." In order for an articulator to work, we had to discover the axis around which the jaw rotated. Then we could put plaster casts of a patient's teeth on this instrument and build suitable replacements.

> WE HAVE COME A LONG WAY, BUT MOST
> DENTISTS ARE STILL PRACTICING "ONE-TOOTH
> DENTISTRY."

So when we did this, the knowledge of the correct treatment for TMJ began. The next step was to identify and name the types of bites and the adverse forces surrounding them.

CENTRIC OCCLUSION OR MAXIMUM INTERCUSPATION (CO)

When the teeth close together in their best fitting position, we call this best bite "centric occlusion" or sometimes "maximum intercuspation." Remember that this term only refers to the fit of the teeth, not to their relationship with where the condyle is located in the TM joint. Even with centric occlusion, in other words, the condyle of the mandible could be part way out of its socket or it could be off center to the right or left.

CENTRIC RELATION OR CENTRIC JAW RELATION (CR)

This term refers to the jaw joint position, not to the fit of the teeth. It is sometimes referred to as "centric jaw relation." It means that the mandible is seated in its rearmost hinge position, not to the right or left but right in the center. It doesn't say anything about how the teeth fit together or how far apart the teeth are. You can have centric relation with your mouth halfway open.

CENTRICALLY RELATED OCCLUSION (CRO)

This is the term that combines the other two terms. The jaw closes to the maximum intercuspation with the jaw in its rearmost hinge position. This position is the main part of the requirements for organic occlusion and is the goal of TMJ treatment. It is mostly disputed by "mainstream" dentists but embraced by gnathologists. It is rarely found in the natural mouth. Almost all the patients seen by dental professionals have a combined average 1.25 mm (+ o r - 1 mm) slide from centric relation to centric occlusion. This slippage in the average person is a predisposing cause of TMJ problems. Gnathologists agree that this slippage (CR to CO) is the first consideration to fix when treating TMJ problems.

THE MOST FREQUENTLY USED PROCEDURE BY GNATHOLOGISTS TO TREAT TMJ IS OCCLUSAL CORRECTION.

OCCLUSAL CORRECTION

The most frequently used procedure by gnathologists to treat TMJ is occlusal correction. This procedure starts with a proper diagnosis. After a proper history, radiographs, tomograms, and complete explanations, models of a patient's teeth are taken. A facebow is taken to relate the upper model to the TM joints on an articulator and a CR wax bite to relate the lower model to the upper model. This relationship is necessary to record so that a correction can be made on the plaster models to ensure the correction can be made properly in the mouth itself. These models are then shown to the patient and kept for the patient's records before any treatment is started. The correction on the tops of the teeth removes interferences to the correct fit of the teeth to coincide with the rearmost hinge position (CO = CR). (Refer to figure 30.) This involves tiny amounts of tooth structure removal. It is 90 percent painless because it only involves enamel. Enamel covers the tops and sides of the crown. It is thickest (about 1 ½ mm) on the tops of the tooth and tapers down to meet the root of the tooth at the gum line. Very occasionally we penetrate the enamel where there are heavy wear spots and could be sensitivity. Chemical agents can desensitize those spots or, if necessary, local anesthesia is used. Then, when the adjustments are finished, a small filling can be placed to prevent decay or sensitivity.

There exists today some disagreement about the sequence of tooth structure removal. Dr. C.E. Stuart in his book *Gnathologic Tooth Preparation* recommends starting with protrusive interferences removal, then lateral interferences next and centric interferences last. I and others find too much tooth structure

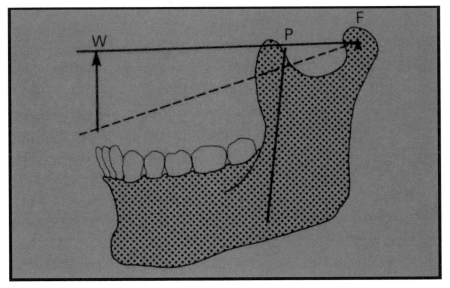

FIGURE 32: *"W" represents work, "P" represents power, and "F" represents fulcrum. The dotted line moving up to the solid line represents the jaw moving up as it chews. This assumes there is no interference and represents a class 3 lever system.*

is lost with this approach. Centric relation should be done first to avoid this problem. If there is doubt in the operator's mind, duplicate models should be taken and the process done both ways to determine which is best.

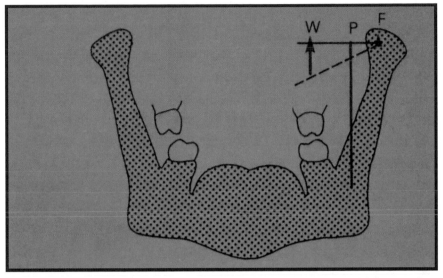

FIGURE 33: *The jaw in the coronal plane shows the class 3 lever system.*

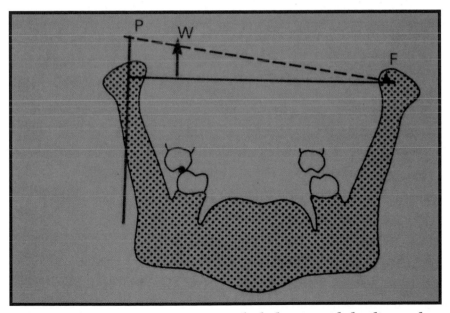

FIGURE 34: *A premature contact on the balancing side leads to a class 2 lever system.*

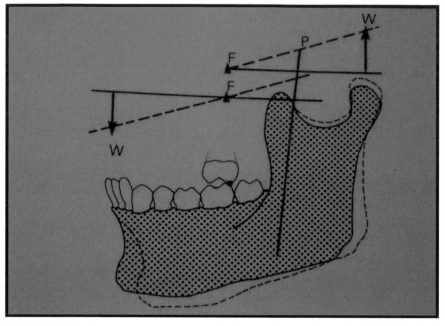

FIGURE 35: *A premature contact in the molar region causes the molar to become the fulcrum. The class 3 lever system distracts the condyle and places harmful pressures on the teeth and TM joint.*

Notice in the diagrams shown in figures 30, 31, 32, and 33 that the leverage systems explain why we need to correct the bite to protect not only the teeth but the TM joints. I want to acknowledge and thank Jan H.N. Pameijer, DMD, in his book *Periodontal and Occlusal Factors in Crown and Bridge Procedures* (1985) for these diagrams. Without knowing these engineering principles diagramed here, it would be difficult to explain why the bite does indeed depend on the TM joint and vice versa. I think figure 35 is the most significant illustration of the ill effects of a slipped bite. The tooth that interferes could act like the olive pit I spoke about earlier. The fulcrum placed on the tooth changes its normal location from the TM joint. Study figure 34 and notice how the lever system changes to a class 2 system, a more powerful one. If the mouth is in centric relation and the teeth have no interference, as in figure 32, then the mechanism functions properly.

Occlusal correction is the first and most frequently used solution in treating TMJ problems. By this name you should get the main idea. We are going to correct the occlusion or fit of the teeth. We are going to change it to coincide with the rearmost hinge point of the jaw. We are going to align the front wheels of your automobile before we put on new tires, so to speak. It is the main way to change the entire bite to harmonize with the TM joints. When you close your teeth together, they guide themselves into a position that is repeatable every time you close your teeth. This position is called, as explained in chapter 3, centric occlusion. This position is where you swallow and close together. The teeth are together when you clench in anger. They are together a lot. It is stated by some experts that they are together for a total of about twelve minutes a day in a healthy mouth. Naturally, there is no other position where they spend this amount of time together. This position when the teeth are together produces a posture in the jaw joints. Unfortunately, this is the ingredient that can cause strain on the joints if it doesn't harmonize with the anatomical best location for those joints. In most folks the jaw joint and teeth don't line up perfectly. You must remember that the "rearmost" position is the correct position, as I have already pointed out, so that is where we must calibrate the teeth. The "occlusal correction" procedure was designed to do just this. We are making the best position of the teeth fit the best position of the TM joints. In other words, "centric occlusion" is the same place as "centric relation."

NOT TAUGHT IN DENTAL SCHOOLS

I did not learn this difficult procedure in dental school. I wasn't even aware of it until 1980. So during my first thirty years I was successfully practicing dentistry, not knowing that there was something I could do to improve how my patients' teeth came together. Actually, there were occasions when I knew something was wrong with a person's bite, but I didn't have a clue how to fix it. There were a few failures of one kind or another that I couldn't explain. That was very distressing to me, and it laid the groundwork for my desire to learn gnathology.

HOW OCCLUSAL CORRECTION IS USED

A TMJ patient, after filling out his or her history and other forms, tells me as best as he or she can the whole story of the problem. My job is to listen and make notes. Then, I do a brief discovery examination. I take a set of dental impressions, a face bow to locate the upper teeth to the articulator, and a centrically related wax bite to locate the lower plaster model to the mounted upper model. I pour the impressions with a quick setting stone (a type of hard plaster) and then trim and mount the study casts on a machine, called an articulator, that duplicates how the jaws move. (see figure 29 on page 81)

In about forty-five minutes, I can show the patient how the bite is aggravating the TM joint. I can then show on the second set of mounted models the way I need to change the surfaces of the teeth to make them harmonize with the correct rearmost location of the jaw (see figure 30), which may take another forty to sixty minutes. Then, I give the patient a booklet to read on the procedure so he or she can go home knowing how we correct the malocclusion. In the quiet of the patient's home, with his or her spouse and the booklet, an informed decision can be made about whether to proceed.

THE NEXT APPOINTMENT

The next time I see the patient, I set the appointment for three hours. I like to check the patient's knowledge of the booklet to make sure the person understands what I'm going to do. It is important to change the bite completely in one appointment to avoid leaving the patient with a bite worse than it was originally. It is possible to produce more pain than the person had to start with. As I explain to the patient, the closer I get to the right bite, the more the teeth touch each other wrong. This can magnify the problem. So we slowly and carefully change the bite by grinding the tops of the teeth. We start by placing the jaw in the rearmost position and gently closing it together on carbon paper. Small grindings are made to begin the removal of unwanted tooth structure or filling material. The time spent doing this is less than you might expect.

IT IS IMPORTANT TO CHANGE THE BITE COMPLETELY IN ONE APPOINTMENT TO AVOID LEAVING THE PATIENT WITH A BITE WORSE THAN IT WAS ORIGINALLY.

Actually, most of the time is spent calibrating which spot is next to be removed, then checking how much to remove. I always enhance the anatomy instead of flattening it. In other words, we produce ridges and grooves rather than just flattening the tops of the teeth. Flat teeth do not work! They mash the food with difficulty but don't chew it.

I always make the changes on models first to show the patient and so that I have a guide as I am working. I always make two sets of original models so I can alter one set to a perfect bite and have the other one to keep showing the original malocclusion.

THE DOWNSIDE OF THE PROCEDURE

People are always concerned that they may lose some of their precious enamel—and well they should be, because we are removing slight amounts here and there to improve the fit of the teeth. The spots of enamel that are removed prevent the jaw from being in its normal rearmost posture. As you might expect, a lot of times some of the material removed is filling or crown material, not enamel. And I am always asked whether it hurts. Rarely do we penetrate the outer protective coat of the enamel. Underneath the enamel is the bulk of the tooth, called "dentin." This is the part of the tooth with feeling. If it is necessary to remove that much enamel, then anesthesia is used and possibly a small filling is placed to seal that area from decay. This procedure is necessary less than 2 percent of the time. Normally, the enamel covering the top chewing surface of the tooth is about one and a half mm thick. The amount of enamel removed in this process is about one or two tenths (0.1–0.2 mm.) of a millimeter. When more than this amount is removed, usually it's because the teeth are very badly aligned with the TM joints. Lots of times in mature dentitions, the resulting sensitivity is so reduced that anesthesia isn't necessary. How to proceed is determined before the procedure starts on a case-by-case basis.

For example, if we left this obstructive tooth structure, theoretically it would wear out anyway. I like to explain to my patients that we actually conserve tooth structure by scientific removal of small amounts instead of letting the mouth wear large amounts with the wrong bite. The mouth will not wear itself "in"; it will wear itself "out." Lots of times there are spots where the enamel is already worn off. Often, we actually take off some of the inner tooth structure (dentin) when the wear pattern is severe on those teeth. Almost always these areas are not sensitive. The body has a marvelous ability to repair itself.

Even the teeth can seal the sensitive areas, given the right body chemistry. Almost everyone has some gum line areas where the enamel is worn away with improper tooth brushing, and they aren't even aware of it. The areas where the enamel is gone can usually be treated with topical agents to relieve any sensitivity. We have several effective chemical agents that can be applied to these areas if necessary. Occasionally, we have to restore teeth completely with crowns, but these cases really fall into the third category of full mouth reconstruction. There are cases that do not fall clearly into one category or another but overlap. The vast majority of treatable cases are done with occlusal correction, probably 80 to 90 percent.

BONDING AND CROWNS WITH OCCLUSAL CORRECTION

Frequently, an occlusal correction case needs an addition to a tooth to bring it up to perfect occlusion. The most important tooth to contact at the same time as the other is the cuspid. As stated before, after removing interference in the posterior teeth, our goal is having both cuspids touch equally along with all posterior teeth simultaneously. Usually one cuspid will touch first as we gradually remove posterior interference. If the anterior teeth also couple when one cuspid touches, we should not take all the teeth down just to satisfy one cuspid that is not touching. At this point we add to the one cuspid that is low. It is vital to the case that both cuspids touch equally. It is a waste of tooth structure to take all of the teeth down to accommodate the one missing canine or cuspid. If all the teeth are settled in to their most stable locking fit and just one cuspid does not hold Mylar shim stock, we prefer to build up that one cuspid.

OUR GOAL IS HAVING BOTH CUSPIDS TOUCH
EQUALLY ALONG WITH ALL POSTERIOR TEETH
SIMULTANEOUSLY.

This addition can be done in several ways, depending on the particular set of teeth. Usually adding some of the new composite material bonded right on to the lower cuspid is all that is necessary. If the particular mouth has a very misplaced cuspid, then sometimes a crown is necessary because the bonding material won't hold up long enough. Sometimes we bond temporarily to produce organic occlusion, then we continue to add to that same spot as the bite settles in and changes to a more stable situation. We can then crown the tooth for a more permanent job. The bonding material used now is very durable and can be matched to the color of the natural tooth very well.

Occasionally, we have to add to some other tooth. The next most likely tooth addition is to the upper or lower incisors so that when the jaw slides forward, those teeth smoothly separate the posterior teeth in a "protrusive excursion." This forward slide is necessary for a patient to bite into a sandwich. Suffice it to say all of the principles of organic occlusion must be installed or the procedure should not be commenced.

ORTHODONTIC TREATMENT

Orthodontics is the next most frequently used treatment for TMJ problems. If the teeth don't line up close enough to do occlusal correction, then orthodontics would be necessary. I would also use the occlusal correction procedure on a finished adult orthodontic case because the teeth are usually worn improperly with the original wrong bite. This correction is usually very minor and is done about three months after retainers are placed.

For TMJ cases, the movement of teeth almost always starts to relieve the pain just by loosening the teeth. This cushioning effect is enhanced by the changing of the habitual wrong bite. These factors must be understood so that the patient doesn't get the wrong idea that his or her treatment is finished. Only when organic occlusion is installed and stabilized with proper follow-up treatment can the orthodontics be successful. These cases represent only a very small minority of TMJ cases.

ONLY WHEN ORGANIC OCCLUSION IS INSTALLED AND STABILIZED WITH PROPER FOLLOW-UP TREATMENT CAN THE ORTHODONTICS BE SUCCESSFUL.

The case in the figures below needed orthodontics to bring the drifted teeth together to ready the case for surgery. After surgery some minor orthodontics was necessary.

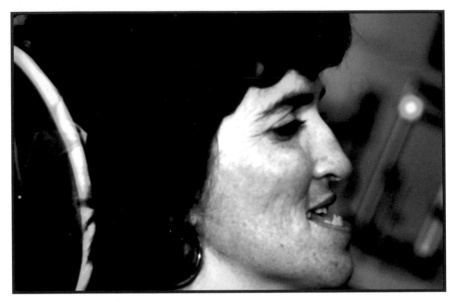

FIGURE 36: *Before jaw surgery*

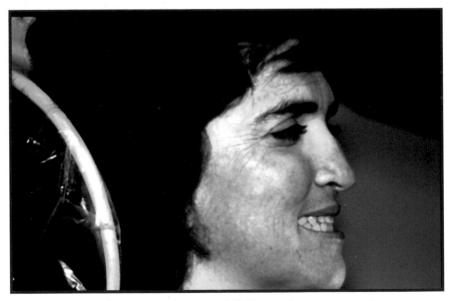

FIGURE 37: *After jaw surgery and full mouth reconstruction*

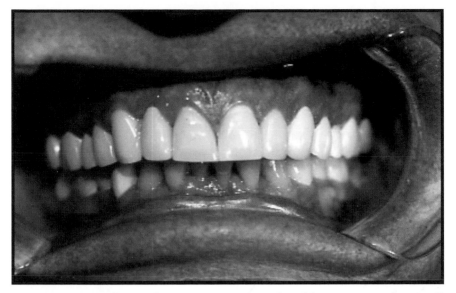

FIGURE 38: *Full mouth reconstruction with gold castings and crystolbal facings*

FULL MOUTH RECONSTRUCTION

"Full mouth reconstruction" is a frequently used way to make the existing teeth harmonize with the TM joint. Often the existing dentistry has been worn badly. The anatomy is gone from the tops of the teeth from the wear caused by a "slip bite" (i.e., the teeth are not aligned with the TM joints). Missing and drifted teeth, broken teeth, and periodontal problems all contribute to the diagnosis. Often bruxism is involved to accelerate the normal wear factor.

Figure 39 shows the extreme wear caused by bruxism in a twenty-eight-year-old male. He couldn't remember when he started to grind. I mounted his models and waxed the worn teeth to their original shapes, hoping to find a reason that he made this grinding effort to obtain a bite that was comfortable. Sure enough his teeth were misaligned in the front, so he couldn't disclude properly. This subconscious irritation caused him to grind. Reconstruction was his only answer.

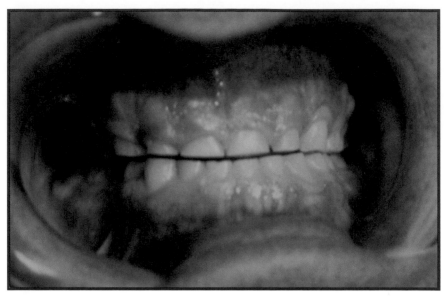

FIGURE 39: *Bruxism*

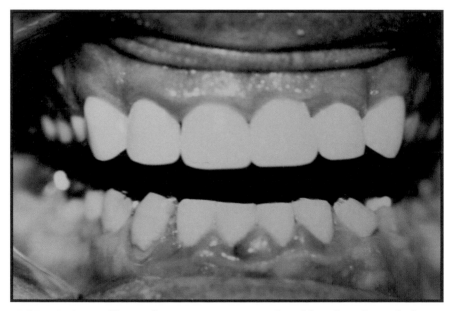

FIGURE 40: *Full mouth reconstruction with gold occlusals and plastic facings. When properly adjusted, the patient stopped grinding.*

Unless gold is used (covered with plastic), the case can fail. The work should be done on a Stuart articulator with precision fit to the bite; otherwise, the patient would start to grind again. This happened several times due to the settling and retreat of the TM joints. Each time I remounted and corrected the slight interferences, his grinding would stop because he could feel the comfort when he bit down. At the time of his treatment, porcelain would have been impossible to calibrate to the accuracy necessary to prevent bruxing. His powerful overdeveloped masseter muscles demanded the highest degree of accuracy, only obtained by casting gold occlusals according to the P.K. Thomas Manual.

CHAPTER 7

History of Gnathology

WHEN DENTISTS BEGAN working many years ago, the majority of the time teeth were extracted because of disease. Now, with the advance of knowledge and technique we can not only save most of the teeth but also restore missing teeth with implants and beautify the existing natural ones. Gnathology goes beyond all these developments by utilizing the engineering principles of our teeth and jaws. There are tiny ridges and grooves on the cusps and fossae of every tooth. We used to look at them and wonder why they all had a certain shape and direction. Now we know, and this area of knowledge is gnathology.

GNATHOLOGY GOES BEYOND ALL THESE DEVELOPMENTS BY UTILIZING THE ENGINEERING PRINCIPLES OF OUR TEETH AND JAWS.

HARVEY STALLARD, PH.B., PH.D., DDS, D.SC.HON.

There were three main original pioneers, and Dr. Harvey Stallard, an orthodontist from San Diego, California, was the principal writer for the group. His life spanned eighty-six years from 1888 to 1974. He started his orthodontic career as a graduate of the Edward H. Angle, M.D., DDS School of Orthodontics, where he followed the same non-extraction philosophy for his entire practice. Dr. Stallard, thanks to

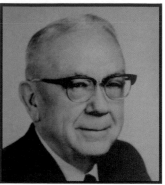

FIGURE 41:
Harvey Stallard, DDS

Dr. Robert Mercer, who recommended him to me, straightened my second daughter's teeth. I was privileged to know him personally, before I became a gnathologist. His genius in language and dental engineering had a profound and beloved effect on all of us in gnathology. Dr. Harvey Stallard actually was the co-inventor of the gnathoscope, the precursor to the instrument we presently use, working separately and cojointly with Dr. McCollum and Dr. Stuart. Dr. Stuart then improved this first attempt in plastic to its present design machined in metal. I, for one, will never forget Dr. Stallard. His writings are our bible of gnathology.

BEVERLY B. MCCOLLUM, DDS

Dr. McCollum was the first of the three pioneers who had a drive for perfection that brought him high honors from the dental profession. His pursuit of knowledge of the mouth led him to make major discoveries that became the basis for organic occlusion. He was born in 1883, graduated from University of Southern California Dental School in 1907, and rose in his profession to accomplish major reconstruction cases before some of the current concepts in gnathology were even discovered.

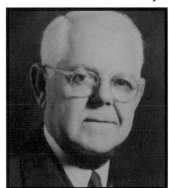

Dr. McCullum's drive and expertise led him to be recognized as the "Father of Gnathology." One of his famous quotes states, "The mouth and teeth are an organ that is vital to the well-being of the individual." Dr. McCollum and Dr. Stallard were drawn to each other's intellectual capacities and cooperated in many discoveries. Dr. McCollum practiced until 1949 in Los Angeles, when a massive stroke caused his retirement. Dr. McCollum pioneered the development of the device used to locate the true hinge axis of the mandible. His efforts were indispensable to the final development by Drs. Harvey Stallard and Charles E. Stuart of the articulator we now use for all the complicated reconstruction cases. Dr. McCollum authored one of the most stinging messages to dentists that I know:

FIGURE 42:
B. B. McCollum, DDS

Fear of more and newer knowledge is a common attribute of every profession. This fear often becomes an excuse for non-acceptance. Often, this fear is founded, in the uninitiated, upon the results obtained by those who prostitute the principles by attempts to "make it easy." There is no royal road to diagnosis in dentistry. Dentistry is difficult—the more we know about it, the more difficult it becomes. It takes more than the ordinary man or mind to master its difficulties. These difficulties are what set dentistry apart, and the mastery of them could give dentistry its place among the learned professions.

DR. MCCULLUM'S DRIVE AND EXPERTISE LED HIM TO BE RECOGNIZED AS THE "FATHER OF GNATHOLOGY."

Dr. B. B. McCollum's accomplishments can be roughly divided into three groups:

1. Full-time private dental practice in Los Angeles from 1909 to 1949.
2. Advocacy of a philosophy of total oral treatment, something new and unusual in his time.
3. Innovations and improvements in dental technology that led to the creation of the science of gnathology—a milestone in dental progress.

CHARLES E. STUART, DDS

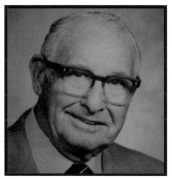

FIGURE 43:
Charles E. Stuart, DDS

Charles E. Stuart, DDS, was the third genius to help fashion our present knowledge of gnathology. Born in 1900, he graduated from University of Southern California Dental School in 1924 and practiced in Ventura, California. He gave us many incredible inventions and a lot of knowledge. His teaching at the USC Dental School early in 1978 was my first exposure to the truth of how the bite works. Even though I had taken other classes from incredibly knowledgeable people in occlusion, he made the subject start to make sense for the first time.

It seemed as though there was a compilation of knowledge out there that would satisfy everyone but took no conclusive stand. It tried to satisfy everyone but didn't tell the real truth, somewhat like what some politicians try to do today. Dr. Stuart was like a breath of fresh air, explaining and demonstrating these principles so that they were at last clear. There were no lingering doubts, no wondering what he meant, no indecision, just complete truth.

This instrument, shown in figure 44, is the only one capable of accurately, consistently reproducing the movements of the human mouth. Dr. Stuart's recording device measures and transfers the information to his instrument so that it can be set to work like the mouth.

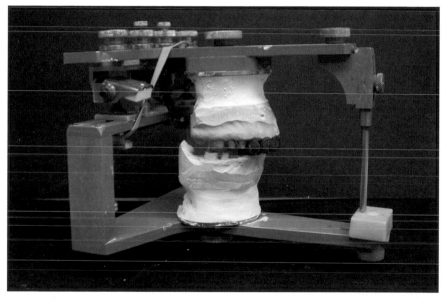

FIGURE 44: *Stuart articulator*

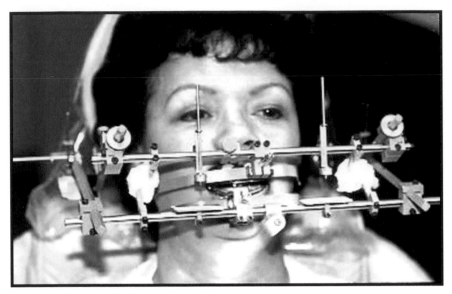

FIGURE 45: *Patient with Stuart recorder*

There are other instruments that claim such distinction and come very close but never quite do all that the Stuart instrument does. When the subject of jaw joint position came up, there was no doubt what the answer was compared to the previous teaching I had had. I took all the courses from Charlie that I could and some of them twice. I even had him, his lovely wife Margaret, Gus Swab, and his love, Connie, and my wife in our home for dinner shortly before his death in 1982. I will never forget asking this marvelous human being a question and his answer. "In all the classes that you have given all over the world, how many of the dentists go back to their offices and actually put into practice what you have taught them?" His answer without hesitation was, "One in ten!" Consider for a moment that only one in ten dentists probably ever took any of his courses, so that means that about one in a hundred ever made the change to gnathology.

What a pity. But of course it would mean great changes in the delivery systems. For example, instead of just preparing that broken tooth with a crown, the dentist would have to take the time to explain that he or she first needed an occlusal analysis. Determining why the tooth broke in the first place depends on studying the bite that the patient brought into the office. This procedure would likely be foreign to the average patient because it depends on an advance in knowledge. Any time we replace teeth or parts of teeth in a worn system, we sew the seeds of destruction.

Dr. Charles Stuart was truly an inventive genius. One of his most newsworthy accomplishments was the development of a radio transmitter then built by Hughes Aircraft to be shipped to Free China in 1946. It was to be used by the army of Generalissimo Chiang Kai-shek to communicate with the U.S. while China was at war. Dr. Stuart was honored with the highest award from the Chinese Republic, the victory medal. The only other person to receive it was General Chennault of the Flying Tigers.

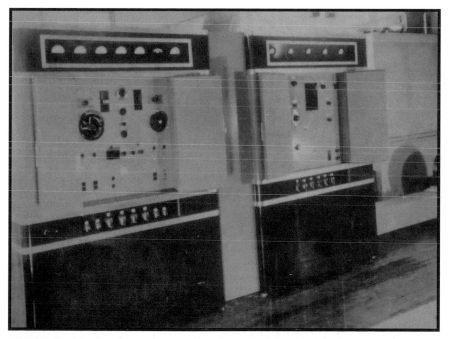

FIGURE 46: *Radio transmitter designed by Dr. Stuart and built by Hughes Aircraft. It was shipped to China in 1946.*

Dr. Stuart spent a year in Shanghai in 1946 engineering the installation of this transmitter and the antenna system and teaching the Chinese how to operate it. It became the fastest automatic intercontinental radio-telegraphic system in the world.

PETER K. THOMAS, DDS

An example of a true gnathologist was the famous dentist Peter K. Thomas. His patients, including Marilyn Monroe, his incredible ability to hold an audience, and his study clubs worldwide made his reputation. He had charisma like no one else in dentistry. He began his high school career as a football star in San Diego and as a graduate of USC opened his practice in Hollywood. He taught and perfected one of the most necessary parts of gnathology, the drip wax technique, originated and taught by Dr. Everitt Payne, a dental technician who was employed by Dr. Thomas and later became a DDS

Dr. Thomas modified his technique and called it "cusp-fossa." It then became known as the PKT wax-up technique. This work trains the dentist to take two opponent arches of prepared teeth in plaster models, place them on an articulator, and flow melted wax on to the plaster teeth to form the natural shapes of original teeth so that they can be cast into gold and used to replace the biting surfaces of the teeth. All of this shaping of wax is accomplished by small additions or "drips" of wax on the prepared surfaces of the teeth to reproduce the organic occlusion that we have been talking about. This is one of the most critical parts of the reconstruction processes. Over the years I have talked and lectured about gnathology, and Peter K. Thomas, DDS was probably the most well-known name that I mentioned. He had study clubs in Europe, Asia, and South America as well as in the U.S. One of the most memorable quotes from this man was, "You must learn to choose the hard right, rather than the easy wrong." Translating this into dental practice, he was saying that the extra work involved to use gnathological instrumentation and knowledge to make a crown was a lot better than simply placing a new crown onto a wrong bite (which would make it worse). This warning by Dr. Thomas was largely ignored by many who attended his lectures. Dr. Thomas was one of the most vocal supporters of Drs. McCollum, Stallard, and Stuart as he spread the good news of gnathology. He was a strong advocate of "learn by doing" and was known as the ambassador of gnathology.

"YOU MUST LEARN TO CHOOSE THE HARD RIGHT, RATHER THAN THE EASY WRONG."

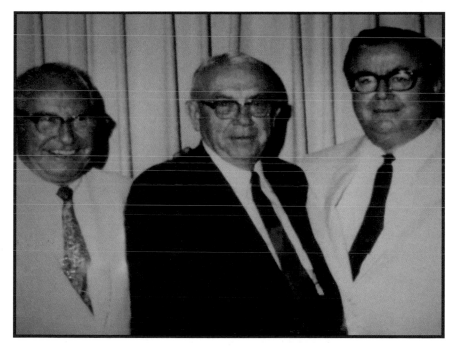

FIGURE 47: *C.B. Stuart, DDS; Harvey Stallard, DDS; P.K. Thomas, DDS*

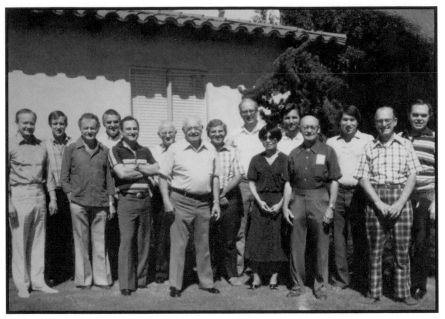

FIGURE 48: *Charles B. Stuart, DDS, wax-up course taught in 1980 at Dr. William Sayre-Smith's office at 4ᵗʰ Ave, San Diego, CA.*
Participants from left to right: Phil Taylor (author), USC '50; Bruce Mullen, USC '67; James Benson, Michigan '55; Art Austin, P&S '49; Irwin Soble, USC '52; Doug Fulton, Penn '54; Charles Stuart, USC '24; Mike Kelley, USC '72; Ron Jones, Baylor '75; Ellen Miyashiro, Oregon '71; Rick Mohrlock, UCSF '75; Gus Swab, USC '40; Barry Aller, USC '71; Bill Sayre-Smith, USC '41; David Schweitzer, Oregon '71.

GUSTAV SWAB, DDS

Gus Swab, my teacher, mentor, and inspiration, will live in my memory forever. He was the fifth genius in gnathology who should be remembered for his devotion to the strictest of adherence to gnathological principles. I used to say that he took no prisoners. "Compromise" was not in his vocabulary. The five volumes by Harvey Stallard, B. B. McCollum, and Charles Stuart, titled *Oral Rehabilitation and Occlusion*, edited by Ben Pavone, were always part of his teaching. They were followed by showing completed cases he had treated. You couldn't help but learn a great deal about treating patients with gnathology at each meeting. He led the Stuart Gnathology Study Clubs for about fifty-six years. He also had study clubs in Los Angeles and Ventura for all those years.

I first met Gus in San Diego in the 1960s when I was in his building (B of A downtown S.D.) and for some unknown reason stopped in to say "hello." He was very polite to show me his office and some of the lab work he was doing. I recall being so dismayed at what he was doing that I had to block it out of my mind. There was no way at the time I could comprehend what he was doing.

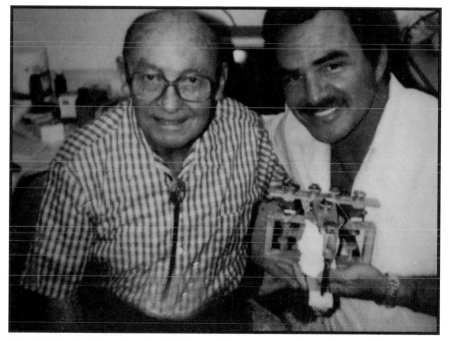

FIGURE 49: *Gus Swab, DDS, with his patient Burt Reynolds*

Gus was a graduate of San Diego High School in about 1935 when my father was the boys' vice principal of that school. Gus never let me forget how my dad gave the students a bad time about smoking in the halls or being late to class. In those days (1930s), those were the common problems and rarely like anything we have today (guns, drugs, etc.). I remember doing a complete mouth reconstruction some years later, and because I didn't know how to do it, I prepared a few teeth at a time and put the crowns back in the mouth a few at a time (maintaining the existing bite). Fortunately, I didn't have a large discrepancy between the correct jaw position (CR) and the tooth position (CO), so I didn't have to change the bite at all. I do remember using the correct jaw position to get the final result, and success was mine. Little did I know how little I knew, and the patient of course didn't either. My thinking at the time was that what Gus was doing was not necessary.

This occurrence probably kept my learning gnathology at bay for quite a while but probably also helped plant the seeds of curiosity. Another patient who needed replacements for several teeth in a row came to me, so I made a long span bridge to fill the gap. Of course, not knowing that his bite was off, the bridge failed and so did the partial denture that I built, without charge, to replace it. This process took a couple of years but served to increase the curiosity about what Gus was doing. This happened about the time TMJ was beginning to become more prominent.

I started to teach one day a week at USC dental school, which again pushed me closer to the fact that I didn't know anything about the bite. So after five years of teaching at USC dental school I was ready for another meeting with Gus Swab. I had purchased a very sophisticated articulator that I eagerly wanted to show Dr. Swab. He invited me to join his study club in late 1979, when we met at Dr. Sheldon Brocket's home for a century club meeting. I remember being excited about this new toy I was trying to use and wanting to learn more about it. I became a member of that study club practically the next day. Then and there my life changed. I had gone far enough into this new discipline to start to become acquainted with at least some of the language, and there was no turning back. Gus taught gnathology and brought me out of the dark. What I'm writing now mostly comes from Dr. Gus. Much of his teaching came from the actual cases he had done. He showed and talked about how the destruction had taken place in the mouths of his patients and the remedies he had constructed. Gradually, I seemed to come into the light about what organic occlusion is, how to diagnose it, and how to obtain it.

MUCH OF THE KNOWLEDGE CAME FROM TRIAL AND ERROR.

Some time ago I asked Gus when he started to treat his patients with organic occlusion. He told me that the full concept of organic occlusion became a reality about 1960. This answer surprised me, because the Stuart instrument came into existence in 1957. He has one of the first production models; I believe it was labeled "#1." But the important information to note is that the knowledge of the reproduction of the mouth onto an instrument came before the full realization of the occlusion knowledge. Parts of organic occlusion were used first before other parts. I believe centric relation (CR) was first. During that phase the belief in "group function" took the place of immediate anterior disclusion. Group function would include some of the posterior teeth in the discluding function. Actually, group function happens after there is considerable wear of the canines. In other words, it is wrong and a result of wear and breakdown of the proper occlusion. So organic occlusion was discovered gradually.

Much of the knowledge came from trial and error. The Stuart fully adjustable instrument contributed much by accelerating the discovery process. Now dentists could put the models on this instrument and set the machine to do what the patient's jaws did. Now they could look inside the mouth with the mouth shut and watch what happened to the cusps and grooves. By comparing the wear of one mouth with another, different one, they could tell what worked the best. After the total concept was arrived at, the benefits proved its validity. According to Gus, balanced occlusion was horrible and caused great pain with many patients whereas organic occlusion brought great relief with all patients.

In other words, *it works*.

I personally want to thank Dr. Gus Swab for saving me from the ignorance, lethargy, complacency, and boredom of ordinary "one-tooth" dentistry.

CHAPTER 8

Occlusal Correction Treatment with Accuracy: The Final Criterion

---

IN DENTAL SCHOOL we were taught that the ultimate goal of a filling was measured at its margin. The way the instructors tested your work was to take a sharp pointed instrument called an "explorer" and run the point over the edge of your filling. If it clicked, the work had to be done over. This click was unacceptable because it meant that bacteria could lodge and grow in that crevice and cause decay. We had this goal of unclickable margins so firmly in mind that we ignored the fit of the bite.

When I was in dental school, occlusion was a relatively minor subject. Actually, organic occlusion wouldn't even be discovered for another ten years. Occlusion was usually mentioned only in conjunction with the fabrication of a complete set of dentures or false teeth. The department of prosthetics (false teeth) believed that the best way to make dentures was with "balanced occlusion." Of course, we now know that organic occlusion works whereas balanced doesn't. The point is that dental schools still emphasize the importance of accuracy of the fit or margins (and I don't disagree with this). But occlusion is still relegated to a lesser priority than margins. If we all knew and agreed that occlusion was the primary cause of TMJ, then we could take a giant leap forward in the dental schools. But that is not yet the consensus position. Malocclusion is not recognized by some dentists as a factor in TMJ complaints.

> WE HAD THIS GOAL OF UNCLICKABLE MARGINS SO FIRMLY IN MIND THAT WE IGNORED THE FIT OF THE BITE.

Accuracy of the bite is top priority in my office and has been for twenty-eight years. Patients are drawn to gnathology and the correction of the bite because of the evident lack of knowledge in most offices and the referral system.

WHAT IS A MICRON?

A millimeter is one thouand microns. A millimeter is also 1/25.4 of an inch, or you could say there are 25.4 millimeters in an inch. A millimeter is about the thickness of a pencil lead. The thickness of a human hair is about 50 microns or .05 mm.

In gnathology, we use a little thin piece of "tinselly" paper called Mylar shim stock. The manufacturer claimed it was .0005 inches thick or one half of a thousandth of an inch. I didn't disbelieve this claim, but I really wanted to find out for myself. I called the hardware store that had been in San Diego since I was a kid and asked for a micrometer. It didn't have one on hand but was able to send to New York for one. Soon I received my Starrett micrometer, made in Athol, Massachusetts, and was able to measure the thickness of Mylar shim stock.

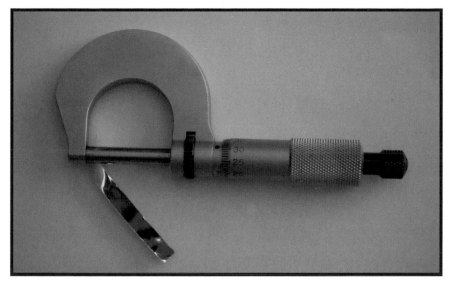

FIGURE 50: *Starrett micrometer with shim stock .0005 inches*

Sure enough, it was 12.7 microns, or .0005 inches, thick. I even doubled it by folding and got .001 inches. I was convinced that what I was doing was correctly interpreted by the Mylar.

When I first watched the use of Mylar shim stock, I had no appreciation at all for what it did. My teacher and mentor Gus Swab demonstrated by holding Mylar in between a patient's teeth in the biting position and tugging on it slightly to see whether the teeth were touching. If that pair of teeth were touching, the Mylar wouldn't move, but if they weren't touching, the Mylar would pull through. So the thinness of the Mylar was an important factor. What we would learn from its use was invaluable for determining which teeth were high and needed to be adjusted, even down to the level of about ten microns. We would test each pair of teeth all around the arch. When we first start the occlusal correction procedure, we don't have to use the Mylar because the teeth that touch first are very obvious to the patient and the doctor. You can actually see the space between the front teeth and part way back on each side. After some of the interferences are removed and the bite closes down, then the Mylar starts to provide much-needed information. During this procedure it is important to hold the patient's jaw in the rearmost position (centric relation). If you don't do this, the patient's muscles will always carry the jaw forward to wherever the teeth fit the best. The muscles have been doing that all the patient's life, so it is perfectly natural for them to keep doing it. We can't expect anything else. Some patients can exert so much force to move the jaw to the old position that we have to push very sternly on their chins. Time after time I have to explain what I'm doing so that patients will cooperate as best they can. I've had a few return the next day with sore chins where I have pushed. This problem should be the only drawback to this procedure.

RELAXING MUSCLES ALLOW RETREAT

When we get close to fitting all the teeth accurately to the new and correct position or posture, then we start to get a correction in the joint itself. We call this healing process "retreat." This shift can be stressful and confusing to the patient and to an inexperienced operating dentist. The patient doesn't know at all that it is happening, and it means more work for the dentist, which is why I recommend at least three hours for the completion of this procedure. I used to think I could do an easy case in two hours or fewer, but I soon learned to allow at least three hours so I didn't have to send the patient home with a transitional bite—i.e., a bite on the way to being perfect but that actually feels worse than the original bite. Actually, it is a new wrong bite. This jaw joint shift is nice, though, because it means we are getting close to the goal and that the muscles are relaxing. With a more relaxed jaw, the job becomes easier, especially on the chin.

WE CALL THIS HEALING PROCESS "RETREAT."
THIS SHIFT CAN BE STRESSFUL AND CONFUSING
TO THE PATIENT AND TO AN INEXPERIENCED
OPERATING DENTIST.

WE NEED THREE HOURS BECAUSE OF RETREAT

There are several schools of thought about this subject. My own thought is that you should always send patients home with the corrected bite. They should be instructed that the bite will change slowly or sometimes quickly as the joint gets used to the new posture. The instructions include return visits for "tune-ups," which are just very small corrections like the major first correction. The usual sequence is about ten returns over about one year. The actual number depends entirely on how much damage has been done to the joint.

The other way is to do as much as you can in about one hour and reappoint in a day or so to finish. This way usually fits better into the dentist's schedule.

The popular consensus is to treat the condition with a splint to reduce or eliminate joint swelling, which would possibly eliminate the need for a lot of "tune-ups" or reappointments. Because of the possible harm that splints do, I prefer the original method. The admonition to obtain "resolution" (retreat) before reconstruction is valid and should always be considered.

CANINES TOUCHING EQUALLY IS OUR GOAL

The canines or cuspids must hold the Mylar at the same time as all the posterior teeth, with the jaw in centric relation and the four incisors barely touching (i.e., the Mylar just barely slides through).

This position must not be controlled by the patient. In other words, the patient must not be using muscles at all to bite down. This difference is gigantic! If the patient bites with any force at all, the teeth that touch first will intrude maybe twenty microns into their sockets, which means that one set that is twenty microns higher than its neighbor will test equally.

MUSCLES MUST BE RELAXED TO TEST THE BITE

But if we get the complete relaxation of the chewing muscles and close the jaw with hand pressure only, the teeth won't sink down and give a false reading. Remember that the periodontal ligaments have different degrees of tightness or looseness depending on the gum tissue health. So the twenty microns I spoke of could actually vary from twenty to fifty microns. Our finished product should be accurate down to about ten microns. I'm totally convinced that some patients can feel differences in height down to about five microns.

THE PRINCESS AND THE PEA

Talk about "the Princess and the Pea"! One of the troubling parts of changing the bite work is that patients who have been living with a bite that is perhaps one quarter of an inch wrong may complain when we correct them to a very good bite that is perhaps twenty microns off. And well they should, because all of a sudden they know what a good bite is. When they started the procedure, only one or two teeth touched wrong; then the slide took place to where all the teeth hit; now sixteen teeth hit just barely wrong, but the patient knows how it feels when everything is just right.

In summary, there are four basic areas of testing the bite with Mylar shim stock: 1) in true centric relation; 2) without any muscle control by the patient; 3) after the major correction is complete; and 4) after the use of a wax bite technique.

BLINDFOLDING THE JAW MUSCLES

When I'm finished with the major correction and am satisfied with the results, I place a wax wafer in between the teeth and, controlling the jaw into centrically related posture, have the patient bite down on the wax. Softly at first, the patient should open and close into the wax at least ten or twelve times or so until the muscles are reprogrammed to this perfect bite; then, the wax should be removed and, very carefully, with the jaw held in centric relation, the jaw should be closed together with either carbon paper or Mylar in between the teeth to test the fit of the teeth and to determine whether they all hit together at the same time in centric jaw relation. All this is done with the dentist's hand on the patient's chin to maintain centric relation. This test is difficult to perform properly and requires some experience to know that it is valid. Only the first try works because the muscles carry the jaw back to the best fit of the teeth immediately. They reprogram themselves by just one or two touches together. The muscles seem to have a very good memory. If you have the wax in between the teeth for a number of closures in centric relation, then the muscles have forgotten the old wrong bite and will close in the relaxed manner you hope to achieve with this correction and follow-ups.

ONLY THE FIRST TRY WORKS BECAUSE THE
MUSCLES CARRY THE JAW BACK TO THE BEST
FIT OF THE TEETH IMMEDIATELY. THEY
REPROGRAM THEMSELVES BY JUST ONE
OR TWO TOUCHES TOGETHER.

We speak of this technique as "blindfolding the muscles." Some patients are much harder to deprogram than others. Most of the time when the occlusal correction is complete the muscles tend to relax because they sense the harmony of the seated jaw socket position (centric relation). One of the things you learn by doing this work is that there are as many variations in terms of patient reactions as there are patients.

I like to explain to my patients that each tooth has maybe one hundred nerve endings under it in its bony socket attached to each root. There could be 439 nerve endings, I really don't know, but for the sake of the discussion we will use one hundred. If you don't believe me that there are a lot, just remember when you bit down on a piece of bone in a hamburger and your jaw "flew open" immediately from the pain. Those little nerves under the tooth were compressed violently and quickly so that the pain pathway was not even in the brain but in a reflex pathway or short circuit causing a reaction that immediately opens the mouth. You don't have to wait till the pain registers in thought and then decide you better open your mouth. No, it happens automatically by reflex. This is, of course, a protective mechanism to keep from breaking a tooth or damaging the gums.

TWO HUNDRED NERVES REGISTER THE WRONG BITE

So if we agree that maybe there are one hundred nerves located under each tooth, then when you bite down and two teeth come together, there are two hundred nerves suddenly activated to tell the brain that this isn't the right bite. So the brain automatically tells the muscles to move the jaw to a better location in which the teeth don't interfere with one another. This allows a better fit for the teeth but a *poorer fit with the TM joint*.

FIT OF THE TEETH ALWAYS WINS

The jaw joint is then a victim of the fit of the teeth. It plays second fiddle to the bite of the teeth. In other words, when there is a choice of fitting the teeth together in their best, most comfortable position and fitting the condyle into the socket in its best most comfortable position, the best fit of the teeth always wins.

Sadly, this fact is very poorly understood, yet it is so necessary to every area of dentistry. Even a high filling can bring about an attack of TMJ. A crown or bridge has an even higher chance of creating TMJ. All sorts of dentistry, including implants, crowns, dentures, extractions, and orthodontia, change the bite and are not considered unusual. But to do an occlusal correction to fit the teeth to the TM joint? Why should that be avoided?

WHEN WE DO ORTHODONTIA, DO WE MOVE TEETH TO A NEW WRONG BITE OR TO THE CORRECT BITE? YOU SHOULD ASK YOUR ORTHODONTIST.

The answer is that organic occlusion is not taught in dental schools and the skill necessary to do an occlusal correction is rare. Are all brain surgeries done in a normal office? Can gnathology become well enough known to help those people with TMJ?

When we do orthodontia, do we move teeth to a new wrong bite or to the correct bite? You should ask your orthodontist. Does he know what organic occlusion is? When you got those expensive implants to fill in where teeth were lost, was your bite corrected first? When you went to your dentist for TMJ and he referred you to an oral surgeon and said you needed open jaw surgery, did he recommend that your bite be fixed first? Do all those expensive X-rays, tomograms, MRIs, and cephalometric tracings provide information that helps with a bite correction? No. What we must always do is take two sets of models mounted on a Whipmix or Stuart articulator in a centric relationship. This gives us in three dimensions (not just two like X-rays) the relationship of the upper to lower jaw with the jaw seated correctly in the socket. Then we know what to do and how to do it accurately.

WALK CAREFULLY ON A SPRAINED ANKLE

Remember, the accuracy you obtain is the key to success. If you have ever suffered a sprained ankle, you didn't dare to bend the ankle at all or the pain would be immediate. Those stretched ligaments wouldn't tolerate the least bit of extra use. If you kept your weight directly down on the foot without any movement to the side, forward, or rearward, the pain would be manageable. Your leg had to be held virtually at right angles to the foot and your weight vertical to the floor. Perhaps this analogy can be applied to the TM joints. The ligaments surrounding each jaw joint are sprained, usually one side more than the other, and we must take away all the strain that we can. This is another reason we know that the rearmost posture is the correct posture for the TM joints. It produces the strain relief necessary to stop the pain. There are very fine dentists with great experience who don't agree with this statement, but if they would take the time to obtain the accuracy necessary to stop this pain, they would agree with me. We are not surgically cutting out diseased tissue. We are not doing physical therapy on the muscles. We are not changing or replacing parts of the jaw joint. We are simply correcting the habitual posture of the jaw joints—the posture that is slightly wrong; the posture that is used every time you speak, chew, or swallow; the posture that controls the engineering of the chewing cycle; the posture that is totally ignored by 99 percent of dentists when they fill or crown your teeth; the posture that isn't taught by most dental schools; the posture that is disputed, argued over, and avoided by most dentists.

NOT A SURE THING

Can we cure TMJ with a bite correction in every case? No. There can be such extensive damage to the structures in the TM joints that surgery is necessary. I personally have referred only one case to an oral surgeon, and it happened to be an arthritic problem. The most non-invasive type of surgery, called "arthrocentesis," was performed with great success. The patient was a known arthritic, and the X-rays showed a remarkable defect in the TM joint. Her bite had been corrected, but the pain remained. This is the sequence of treatment that is commonly reversed. First, the bite must be fixed, then, if there's no relief, surgery may become necessary. On the other hand, I have had many cases that have had joint surgery, and not one of them had the bite fixed.

DESCRIPTION OF A SURGICAL FAILURE

One of the most important examples of surgical failure was a young lady who had both joints operated on and "proplast" laminate implant put into the right joint to replace the natural disc and a minor placation on the left TM joint. This surgery was done in 1983. A second surgery was performed in 1987 with the diagnosis of internal derangement to both left and right joints and supra-erupted tooth #15 (upper left second molar). It is interesting to note that the surgical report mentions a tooth #15 that is too long but fails to mention that anything was done or should be done. This is an admission that the surgeon either failed to fix a problem or that the problem wasn't considered important. My guess is that the surgeon just didn't believe that the posture in the joint was the problem.

The next surgery to the right joint was to remove the proplast implant and replace it with a new implant made of .050 Silastic material. A layer of fat removed from the hip was placed in the joint space. The left joint was again opened, and dense adhesions were removed. After five months of pain and misery, the patient reported to another hospital with this description of her problem: "I've seen over fifty doctors, and I have pain that starts mostly at night with a lightning pain followed by a forward shooting jerk of the head and neck; my jaw opens involuntarily, which awakens me; then the pain starts. After the 'lightning' I feel like something would 'break' inside my head, then the jerk of the head and neck, opening of the jaw, and the headaches."

She had a third surgery in May of the following year with motivation from pain, headaches, difficulty closing her right eye, and very restricted movement of her jaw. She couldn't open her mouth past about one-third of the normal opening. She also couldn't move her jaw to her left side, indicating immobility of her right joint. She couldn't protrude her jaw straight forward to bite with her front teeth without it deviating to her right. It was noted in her surgical report that "there was no stable occlusion" and that there had been two previous surgeries, "neither of which were successful in the remotest sense." She also continued to live with pain and headaches. This third surgery on the right joint removed the previously placed Silastic implant and quite a bit of the original "proplast" implant that remained even after the second surgery had supposedly removed it. A bony ankylosis had started to form at the medial pole of the right joint, which would account for the lack of range of motion.

FOUR SURGERIES DONE WITH GOOD INTENTIONS, BUT SHE STILL HAD NO BITE

A fourth surgery was done to shorten the coronoid process and cut loose the attachment of the temporalis muscle. This operation was designed to allow her jaw more freedom. It seemed to at first, but by the time I saw her, her restrictions were still very great, and the jaw movements only one-third of normal.

All this was done with good intentions (I'm sure) to get her well from pain and jaw restrictions. None of it was successful, though, because the surgeons didn't know that the bite correction procedure would help. They didn't know what a correct bite was. They didn't know how to obtain a correct bite. They did know how to cut her open and cut up her jaw joint. This indeed should be the last resort.

I saw her in April of 1990. She was referred by her boyfriend, whose entire mouth I had rebuilt with new gold crowns and white plastic for looks, replacing porcelain crowns in a bite that had caused him pain. So she had been convinced that correcting the bite did have some possibilities. After mounting models and showing her the very poor fit of her teeth, she urged me to try this new approach to her problem. I explained that I couldn't undo the damage to her joints, but I could take some stress off the joints and let them heal. I then made a very thin gold splint, higher on one side than the other, to allow her bite to be even and correct. This measure provided the first relief of pain she had known since before her first surgery. After this dramatic change and relief, she wanted to make the change permanent. I then rebuilt all the upper teeth. She didn't totally regain full opening of her mouth, but she did improve and was pain free. *Yes, accuracy of the fit of the teeth is the final criterion of success.*

CHAPTER 9

What to Expect after Treatment

YOUR FIRST FEELINGS AFTER THE THREE-HOUR APPOINTMENT

IMAGINE THAT WE have just finished correcting your bite. You find that you can close your teeth together with minimal effort. You notice that when you touch your aligned jaws together, your teeth make a noticeable sound—a louder sound than you were used to. Instead of one or two teeth meeting at one time, now they all contact at once. If you were to clench your teeth together, you would notice that they don't shift your jaw into a different position any more. It feels comfortable. It feels right. You begin to wonder why this correction wasn't made before. You notice that the muscles in your face and around your jaws are relaxed. Your face seems to be normal again. Sometimes you seem to notice your front teeth are touching in places that didn't used to touch. One side seems to be touching together stronger and more readily than it used to. Maybe your gnathologist had to add some bonding to one side or the other to make it even, and the new addition might seem unusual and maybe too high. This feeling is very common, and the newness of it accentuates the awareness. Even though the canine teeth should touch at the same time, most of the time they don't, and so we have to add some bonding material to make them do that. Occasionally the bonding is actually too high and has to be sanded down slightly. When the bite is first calibrated to the new position, it will change very quickly but ever so slightly. This change is what we call *retreat*.

IT FEELS COMFORTABLE. IT FEELS RIGHT. YOU BEGIN TO WONDER WHY THIS CORRECTION WASN'T MADE BEFORE.

RETREAT—THE SHIFT OF THE JAW POSTURE

This shift of the position of your jaw is first felt usually just after you leave the office. I try my best to explain this phenomenon to my patients, but until you actually experience it for yourself, even the best efforts fail. I like to explain it this way: "The bite will feel perfect until you walk out the door, but before you can start your car it will feel wrong." It happens that quickly. Just what happens?

RETREAT—HEALING

The change takes place in the jaw joint itself. Actually, the TM joints themselves change. The bones get closer together. Maybe the disc in between the bones moves into a better place ever so slightly. Maybe there is some swelling in the joint due to the years of wrong posture that goes away. We know that there is muscle relaxation going on because of the corrected bite, particularly the superior head of the lateral pterygoid muscle that is attached to the front of the disc. Also, there is a ligament attached like a rubber band to the back of the disc that pulls the disc back and keeps it on top of the condyle as the mandible returns to its rearmost posture (CR). Maybe it is the relaxation of the forward pulling muscle that has continually kept the disc over the head of the condyle in its abnormal forward posture. Because of that relaxed muscle in front, the overstretched ligament in back gradually returns to normal and pulls the disc backward into a more normal posture.

SWOLLEN TISSUES IN THE TM JOINT

Perhaps the disc itself is swollen and not compressed as much in the new posture, and so with a load in a new place now it has to settle in to its normal compressed state. All or any of these conditions will cause the jaw to move backward and upward very slightly to a new location. This phenomenon we call "retreat." This change takes place only in the TM joints, but it feels like the teeth move and don't fit anymore. Remember that the bite was calibrated down to about 5 to 10 microns. If the perception of the new bite is good, then the perception of the retreat will be equally good (or bad in this case). Remember that a human hair is about 40 to 60 microns thick. This shift is only about one-fourth of the thickness of a human hair. Normally, you wouldn't pay any attention to this amount of shift, but when you have been introduced to a near-perfect bite and have experienced this degree of accuracy, you don't feel right until you get it back. You have literally been spoiled. Whatever happens, we consider it a healing process. It is good, and the quicker it happens, the healthier the joint.

CATEGORIES OF REACTIONS

Everyone's awareness of "retreat" is different. Some folks don't notice much at all by the time they return for a "tune-up." They think they don't need it. Occasionally they don't, but most often they need it just as much as the others but don't perceive the need. These are the lucky ones and fit into the first of three categories. I like to divide the patients into these categories to help me predict the future treatment that will be necessary for them.

> I LIKE TO DIVIDE THE PATIENTS INTO THESE CATEGORIES TO HELP ME PREDICT THE FUTURE TREATMENT THAT WILL BE NECESSARY FOR THEM.

FIRST CATEGORY—THE EASIEST

The first category is the easiest to deal with and heals the quickest. I wish everyone were in this category because then the procedure would be easy to teach and learn. Everyone could have it done, and the success rate would be 100 percent. It could be treated in every office with ease and utilized before normal dentistry was undertaken. These folks usually don't have any symptoms to speak of and don't need many, if any, follow-up treatments. There is no need for extreme accuracy. If a retreat occurred, the patient probably wouldn't be aware of it. These folks are usually easier to work on also. Their jaw muscles are loose and relaxed, making it easier to do the whole procedure.

SECOND CATEGORY—THE AVERAGE

The second category is the largest and most likely to occur. These folks take about a year to complete their treatment of "tune-ups," consisting of about ten return visits spread out over a year or so to correct for the "retreat" and to allow the jaw joint to continue to heal and normalize.

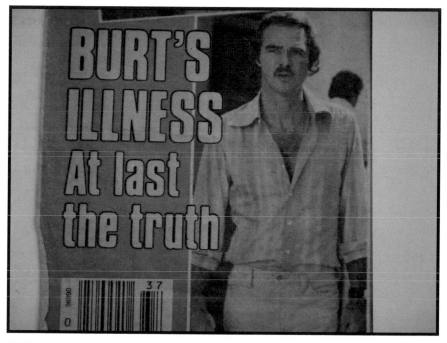

FIGURE 51: *The cover of* Globe, *9 October 1985: Burt Reynolds with TMJ*

BURT REYNOLDS NEARLY LOST HIS CAREER WHEN HE WAS HIT IN THE FACE WITH A CHAIR THAT WAS WROUGHT IRON INSTEAD OF BALSA WOOD. THIS INCIDENT WAS THE "INCITING CAUSE" OF HIS TMJ.

THE BURT REYNOLDS STORY

Burt Reynolds nearly lost his career when he was hit in the face with a chair that was wrought iron instead of balsa wood. This incident was the "inciting cause" of his TMJ. It caused an addiction to Halcion and trips to more than thirty dentists and dental surgeons in an attempt to find help. The accident took place during the filming of *City Heat* with Clint Eastwood in 1984. Reynolds ignored the jaw fracture until he was diagnosed with TMJ, at which point it was found that the old fracture had healed. He was mistreated with splints and capping of all his lower front teeth. Finally, he was referred to my mentor Gus in about 1985.

In his autobiography, *My Life*, Reynolds describes going to the House Clinic in L.A. for the dizziness he suffered and how he had tubes put in his ears to relieve it. Then he found Dr. Gus Swab, who rebuilt his mouth and saved his life from the Halcion addiction that nearly did him in while he was trying to cope with the TMJ.

One prominent dental school cut off his lower front teeth and then capped them to try to help him. None of these attempts by well-meaning but ignorant dentists helped in the slightest. In *My Life* Reynolds explains that every few months he had to return because "my brand-new mouth changed ever so slightly as it settled in. I had to relearn how to bite and chew—how to as they say, find home base" (pg. 282). He was talking here about "CR" or centric relation (what he calls "home base"). He had to come back every few months to correct for the retreat he was experiencing.

Being a student of Dr. Gus and meeting with him every month at his study club, I was privileged to see and hear about the gold remedies that Gus made for Burt Reynolds. After recovery, Reynolds went back home to Florida, where his family lived. He then succumbed to nagging to make his mouth look better and went to a supposed TMJ dentist, who removed all Gus's work and replaced it with porcelain. Less than a year later, Reynolds returned to Gus's office with a dual bite. He had to move his jaw to his left to fit the left side of his new work and then move to his right to fit the right side of his new porcelain crowns together. I actually saw this work and grieved for Reynolds while Dr. Gus started the process of rebuilding his bite. This story, as bizarre as it is, points out that Reynolds's occlusion had to be exact and remain that way for the rest of his life. His fight with TMJ nearly wrecked his career and has become a huge banner for gnathology and accuracy of the bite. Burt Reynolds is a good example of the third category of re-treat (the toughest).

THIRD CATEGORY—THE TOUGHEST

This third category is the toughest and fortunately the least likely to occur. Patients in this category are cursed with an ultra-sensitive nature about most everything and are usually the TMJ cases that everyone else has failed to cure. They probably have worn every conceivable kind of splint without benefit. Some of them have had replacement parts surgically inserted in their TM joints by ignorant dentists. Proplast, Silastic, Teflon, titanium, harvested bone, fat, and who knows what else are used. Burt Reynolds had one dentist recommend an artificial joint, which fortunately he refused. Lots of these patients have had orthodontics along with these other things, but none of them has been told his or her bite needs to be fixed. This is truly strange, particularly given that the orthodontists are supposed to know what a good bite is. In reality, they don't. There are tragic stories I have read about, and I have treated quite a few more such cases. These poor folks don't know where to go for real help. Some patients end up suicidal because of the relentless pain. Most of the folks in this category whom I have treated need from two to seven years of care and adjustments, and a very few need an entire lifetime. The damage to their joints is so extensive that it takes that long to return to normal. It reminds me of the ancient Chinese practice of binding the feet of women because it was considered attractive to have small feet. Some of the pictures of the results of this practice are so grotesque that it is hard to believe anyone would continue to do it. In a much lesser way, the tissues of the TM joint have been bound into the wrong posture by virtue of the malpositioned teeth. The point is that when the tissues are badly deformed for long periods of time, the healing may never be complete.

This Third Category Takes More Effort

This third category requires some careful consideration. When the teeth with their interdigitating cusps force the jaw to an unwanted and antagonistic posture to the TM joints for long enough periods of time, the body builds up compensating fortresses of otherwise unnecessary tissue. This tissue is gradually broken down and disposed of when the corrected bite is installed. The time is different for different degrees of malposture and for different degrees of healing vigor. Many factors enter into the picture. Vitamins, minerals, exercise, sleep, heredity, faith, and emotional health all enter the equation. Every dentition is slightly different, and every malocclusion is different, not to mention the type of dentistry that has been provided to the mouth. A young, untouched set of unworn teeth would guide us more toward orthodontia than occlusal correction by itself. An older dentition with much replacement work would call more for reconstructing the entire bite. The fact remains, though, that the procedure that works most often for the largest number of people is occlusal correction. It is by far the most useful procedure in dentistry today.

THE FACT REMAINS, THOUGH, THAT THE
PROCEDURE THAT WORKS MOST OFTEN FOR
THE LARGEST NUMBER OF PEOPLE IS
OCCLUSAL CORRECTION. IT IS BY FAR THE
MOST USEFUL PROCEDURE IN DENTISTRY
TODAY.

WHEN YOU GO HOME

The feeling of benefit soon diminishes because of the retreat. Both the length of time you have tolerated the malocclusion and the degree of malocclusion correlate with the healing time. I notice that people in the third category often come back even the next day for a "tune-up." Sometimes they have to return three or four times a week for a couple of weeks. This situation is not unusual. The damage is so severe in these cases that a great deal of healing must take place. I always explain that it is good that they have to come back soon because it indicates the healing is taking place quickly. The quicker the healing, the quicker we get done. Now, here is the bad news: The original bite only hit wrong on a few back teeth. So as the retreat takes place, all of the newly calibrated teeth hit wrong. The more teeth hitting wrong now magnifies the problem. That can actually make more pain than a patient had before we started. Only patients in the third category have this problem, fortunately, and only a small percentage of them. The pain level is very difficult to predict. We try very hard to prevent total disillusionment, but in spite of the booklet and a quiz about what is in it, we lose a patient once in a while. These folks are almost all resistant to the truth of healing and what's involved. They are in denial. Probably they have experienced discouragement so often with the different attempts at treatment that when the first bit of pain comes back, they feel like this treatment isn't going to work either. The testimonial stories in the next chapter, though, show that there is always hope.

THE USUAL HEALING SCENE

Most often, after the major three-hour correction appointment, a patient goes home with the first hope he or she has had in years. The person's pain is gone, the face is relaxed, and all the teeth hit at the same time. You may not consider these changes to be too much to brag about, but you would be surprised at how many people haven't had all their teeth hit at the same time for their entire lives.

Most people have a set of teeth that hit fairly evenly but just out of harmony with the TM joints. These are the most likely candidates for the occlusal correction procedure and the most successful cases. In the first month following the procedure and after a couple of "tune-ups" for maybe half an hour of adjustment each, these patients settle into a fairly stable bite that is comfortable, and we only have to see them maybe once a month for a couple of months, then every other month for a couple times. The average case takes about one year and ten "tune-ups." The amount of grinding to remove the interfering tooth structure or filling material is very slight. Most of the time (about 95 percent) is spent measuring and checking to find the spots that interfere with a perfect bite. We show these spots to patients before we even start a case. The patient knows exactly what to expect and understands that there is going to be retreat and follow-up work after the initial treatment.

Some Testimonials

MY LIFE CHANGED *dramatically for the better after meeting Dr. T. After living half my life with constant pain in my face and neck, I finally found a dentist who knew what was wrong with me and how to correct my medical problems.*

It all started when I was thirteen years old and received braces for my teeth. Seven of my baby teeth were removed along with four permanent teeth by my orthodontist in Chula Vista. After three years, yes, my teeth were straight and pretty, but only two back molars on the right side of my mouth would meet when I would bite my teeth together. There was a quarter-inch gap between the other teeth. The only way I could chew my food was to position the food to touch there on the two right back molars. This misalignment of my bite started slowly to give me problems.

AFTER LIVING HALF MY LIFE WITH CONSTANT PAIN IN MY FACE AND NECK, I FINALLY FOUND A DENTIST WHO KNEW WHAT WAS WRONG WITH ME AND HOW TO CORRECT MY MEDICAL PROBLEMS.

When I was nineteen years old, I went to a so-called noted TMJ specialist in Chula Vista with complaints of headaches, neck aches, and constant swelling of the right side of my face. This dentist recommended ice packs, electrical stimulants, and splints. After four months of treatment he proceeded to give me painful cortisone shots in my TM joints.

With no relief in sight, I went to another specialist in La Mesa. This dentist designed a new splint and recommended reconstructive surgery. The dentist went so far as to hire a hypnotist to see if my illness was self-caused. After five months of this I decided to stop treatments and go on a self-help program. I only ate soft foods and liquids. I still suffered with the swollen face, headaches, and a very stiff neck. Sometimes my right hand would fall asleep for days.

At twenty-one years old I was in a bad car accident and was placed in a hospital in the San Diego area for two weeks in traction for a whiplash. A harness was strapped to my chin to pull my neck muscles slowly with weights, but it also aggravated my TM joint problems. I was in constant pain, and my TMJ swelled on the right side of my face. I was sent to a hospital in Los Angles for X-rays taken by a special machine that turns you upside down to see if the jaw hangs open correctly and to see if the pain was caused by the auto accident. An orthopedic surgeon was called in and recommended surgery to replace the TM joints on both sides of my face. I was told that arthritis had caused the joints to deteriorate beyond repair and nothing else could be done to help me.

Again I went on liquids and soft foods for six years. If I would eat so much as an apple, then my face would swell, and I would have to take codeine and go back to the ice packs. I was always in pain but did not feel that I could live with the problems and uncertainty that the TMJ operation would bring.

Then at my husband's urging I went to a TMJ clinic in Escondido. The doctors started with splints, then moved to electrical therapy, then to ice packs. Because of the years of abuse to the TM joints and the splints, my face swelled to four times its size. I lost feeling and strength in both hands and was unable even to open a door. I was sent to a psychologist for analysis to see if my problems were self-caused.

Finally, I was admitted to an Escondido hospital, where a team of five doctors ran a series of tests on me. The doctors thought I had contracted muscular dystrophy, and then they thought I had cancer. An arthritis doctor was called in, and I was told I was suffering from "myo-facia," an inflammation of the tissue that covers the muscles. I was given heat packs, muscle relaxants, and daily massages. I spent seven days in the hospital. I really feel the reason I got better was I refused to wear the splint any longer and went back to a soft food diet.

By my own good luck I then went to see Dr. Taylor in Rancho Santa Fe. He convinced me that all that was wrong with me was that the bite didn't fit—that the dentist who put on my braces did make my teeth straight and pretty but didn't line them up properly for chewing food. The reason the right side of my face had swollen up was because I had been only chewing on the right side, and the muscles on the right were overdeveloped. This was so simple yet so radical to me after hearing half my life that my problems were in my mind or that the TM joints must be replaced.

HE ALSO TOLD ME THAT SPLINTS WERE A WASTE OF TIME AND ARE JUST LIKE A ROCK IN YOUR SHOE–THEY ONLY AGGRAVATE THE PROBLEM.

I felt skeptical and brought my husband with me for my second consultation appointment. Dr. Taylor said it would take about ten months to a year to fix my bite because of the major corrections needed. I would have to come in twice a month. He also told me that splints were a waste of time and are just like a rock in your shoe—they only aggravate the problem. My husband and I so wanted to believe that a treatment of just grinding my teeth to fit would correct my problems. The fee really didn't matter to us; we were so desperate. Dr. Taylor even offered the procedure for free, just to get me out of pain. He told me he was absolutely sure he knew exactly what caused my pain and knew he could correct my bite. But it was Dr. Taylor's sincere concerns for my health and his ongoing dedication to his profession of helping people that convinced me to go ahead with this procedure. He did everything he promised. I feel great and happy, and I will always have a sincere appreciation of Dr. T. for the rest of my life.

G. S.

AUTHOR'S NOTE: She had four bicuspids removed (improperly) for orthodontia at age thirteen and was left with spaces between her front teeth and an open bite. This was a bite that did not allow any teeth to touch except the right back two molars. This created torque on the joints (see chapter 5, figures 34 and 35). She had been misled into believing that the posture in the jaw joints had nothing to do with the suffering she endured. She realized that rest and soft foods were the only thing that helped.

HERE IS THE SUMMARY: *When I was twelve, I was riding a bike, and my friend was sitting behind me. We went down a hill and crashed. She landed on top of me. My front tooth was knocked out and my jaw fractured. A Navy doctor wired my mouth shut for six weeks. When I was fourteen, I had braces put on and some teeth were pulled (four premolars). When I was twenty-three, Dr. C. H. determined that I had a TMJ disorder because I had clicking and pain. He referred me to an orthodontist. The two dentists agreed I should wear a splint. Also, the orthodontist discussed the case with a TMJ specialist and said that my injury was too old to merit oral surgery*

The splint relieved a lot of pain, and the orthodontist slowly weaned me off of it. During my treatment with the orthodontist, sometimes the pain was worse than before when he had put braces on me. Toward the end of my treatment the orthodontist told me my braces would soon be coming off, but I still had pain. My ex-mother-in-law recommended Dr. T. I'm very fortunate that I found Dr. T. Sometimes I meet people who have TMJ disorder and are in great pain even when they are being treated.

Sincerely,
C. B.

AUTHOR'S NOTE: She had X-rays that showed the head of the condyle had broken off and lodged in the space ahead of the glenoid fossa where it healed to the ramus of the mandible. It functioned normally there but was about three-quarters of an inch forward of where it belonged. The socket ligament healed into this abnormal location, which seemed to function normally except there was no "eminence" in front, so that her jaw on the right side went up when she protruded forward and the left (normal) side traveled down the way it was supposed to. This condition created all sorts of problems, not only with orthodontic treatment but also with the chewing cycle. I ended up crowning the lower right canine to make it long enough to function properly because I was unable to raise (extrude) it orthodontically. I achieved organic occlusion, and the second I did her pain was gone. The bite is fairly stable now, requiring "tune-ups" about twice a year. Logic motivated me to install organic occlusion, and it worked.

Dear TMJ Support Group,

I am writing to you in response to a piece I saw on 8-28-94 on American Journal. I too am a TMJ survivor and would like to share my story with your group of the man who saved my life. My battle with debilitating pain began in September of 1989. I was rear-ended in an auto accident. During the next sixteen months I suffered from neck pain, limited neck movement, three-day migraine headaches, ranging from dull to blindingly painful, nausea, vertigo, nosebleeds, blackouts, memory loss, vocabulary loss, and shooting pain in my right eye. I sought help from my family doctor, a chiropractor, two neurologists, an acupuncturist, and a carpal tunnel specialist. I was subjected to every test known to man. Not one of these doctors could find any physical evidence of my injury. One doctor suggested my problem was psychological. Many hard drugs were prescribed to cover up my pain, but no hope of solving the problem was offered. My list of unsuccessful prescriptions includes: Furinol, Codeine, Valium, Darvon, Darvocette, Demerol, Percodan, vitamins, and Chinese tea. Unfortunately, my body has a high tolerance to pain killers, and none was effective. On my own I tried alcohol, vibrators, massage, hot baths, a Jacuzzi, body braces with supports, diet change, blood thinning, and total bed rest. I was desperate.

I WAS SUBJECTED TO EVERY TEST KNOWN TO MAN. NOT ONE OF THESE DOCTORS COULD FIND ANY PHYSICAL EVIDENCE OF MY INJURY.

I should mention that I am an electrician and started my own business in 1986. At the time of the accident I had been married one year and was expecting my first child in one month. I did not have any medical insurance. Needless to say, I was spiraling to my financial ruin, being unable to work more than two days a week.

In January of 1991 a friend recommended a neurologist in San Diego. My first ray of hope came from a drug called Pamelor. At least it shortened the frequency of my three-day migraines. I continued this drug daily for over one year. I did not want to be dependent on this drug for the rest of my life. I tried to wean myself off of it, but I quickly returned to an unacceptable level of pain. I resumed the Pamelor and my search for a cure.

This is where my case takes an exciting and unexpected turn toward my diagnosis and recovery from TMJ. On occasion, I had done electrical work for Dr. T., a dentist in the San Diego area. I knew he was a specialist, but as a courtesy to me he gave my mouth the once over. It had been many years since my last visit to a dentist.

Dr. T. asked if I was having any problems. My first response was, "No, not with my teeth." Dr. T. then explained that my bite was obviously off and that my past dental work had done me more harm than good. I could be experiencing jaw joint pain, headaches, or teeth grinding. I said yes!! I explained my history of pain and symptoms for two and a half years. Dr. T. pulled out a jaw model and explained how whiplash can tighten and strain muscles in the head and neck and cause the misalignment of a person's whole jawbone. I took this news to my neurologist, who quickly discounted my theory of TMJ as a generic term overused by the medical field and as that year's "designer" ailment.

I quit taking the Pamelor, and my pain returned. After a month of suffering I had had enough. I called Dr. T. for an appointment. Plaster casts were made and measurements were taken of my mouth and jaw. After a week of studying my problem, Dr. T. called me to discuss my options. My mouth for the most part had to be rebuilt and my bite readjusted. I quickly agreed. If this man could deliver a fraction of the relief he projected, it would be nothing short of a miracle. Everything he said made sense, and best of all no surgery was necessary. Three days after Dr. T.'s work, I felt such a notice-

able relief that I would have been happy if no other improvement followed. In two weeks I was free of pain and in utter disbelief. In the following months, if I felt a headache coming on, I would run up to the doctor's office and in twenty minutes be back on track. My regular follow-up adjustments lasted about one year. I now see Dr. T. about every six to nine months.

THREE DAYS AFTER DR. T.'S WORK, I FELT SUCH
A NOTICEABLE RELIEF THAT I WOULD HAVE BEEN
HAPPY IF NO OTHER IMPROVEMENT FOLLOWED.
IN TWO WEEKS I WAS FREE OF PAIN AND IN
UTTER DISBELIEF.

I am such a believer in this man's treatment that I sing his praises to anyone who will listen. After watching those people suffering on American Journal *from the effects of TMJ surgery, I know if there is anyone on earth that could help them, it is my doctor.*

The scary part is, had I been diagnosed with TMJ in the beginning, I would have been directed to have surgery too. When you are in such pain, you will grab at straws for relief. I feel surgery should be a last resort for any ailment. More education is needed in the field of TMJ. My healing was totally natural, with no destruction, and was simple—so simple I was skeptical. It was a stroke of luck that I stumbled on to one of the few pioneers who treat TMJ without surgery. I am enclosing a patient guide book I received from Dr. T. I hope you pass this information on to your group. Better yet, I hope this is old news and you already know of his work.

Sincerely,
Brad S.

WELL, YOU BEST KNOW *that I have lost half of my hearing since I was seven from the measles, so when I first heard about "occlusal correction," my imagination went wild! It sounded like Doc Phil was into some kind of occult rehabilitation or some kind of new torture being a D-E-N-T-I-S-T and all. But what a change in life for me at age forty-six! Imagine going through life grinding your teeth, squinting, making weird faces, and people always asking if you were hurt or constipated. Some even had the nerve to offer me their Preparation H! Good God, I hated that.*

When Doc Phil first noticed the faces I was making, I was amazed how quickly he knew why it was happening. Since I didn't have an overbite or under bite but one hell of an uneven bite, Doc Phil said I needed an occlusal correction. He didn't even have the "wait-till-I-get-him-in-the-chair" look.

I told Doc Phil that I had not been to the dentist in fifteen years, that I hated drills, needles, and especially dentists. Boy, did I have some bad experiences! I told him that I even punched one dentist from reflex when he accidentally hit a nerve and how I knew I needed some teeth work when one of my crowns broke off and the root fell out. Doc Phil just smiled knowingly. You know that hypnotic stare that dentists give you before they jump into your mouth.

Next problem was getting up the nerve to sit in that chair. *Well, Doc Phil gave me the incentive and asked if he could demonstrate his process to other dentists that he was teaching. My first thought was four sets of hands probing my mouth—no way, José! Doc Phil assured me that there would be no needles, pain, or ritual torture and that only he would be working in my mouth (sounds* insane) *while the others observed his techniques. He cautioned that the process would take three to four hours. No pain, no needles, no more grinding, no jawbone tension, and no squinting or constipated faces. I'd be eating on the right side of my mouth for the first* time in my life and able to snap my jaw shut without pinching my cheek. Okay. I was actually looking forward to it.

Doc Phil first made a mold of my bite and strapped it into a specially designed vice. Then he showed me the problems I had with my bite and what he would need to do to correct it. Doc Phil has an entire office wall collection from floor to ceiling of his victims' jaws mounted like trophies—shelves of them just staring at you. If they could only talk.

Zero hour. Doc Phil had me relate my problems to his student dentists. I told them that I was told by every dentist I had seen that I had to stop grinding my teeth. One dentist determined that I was grinding my teeth in my sleep and fitted me for a mouth piece to use when I slept. Can you imagine trying to find the damn thing in the morning if it wasn't poking you in the ribs? Then I related that I never completely chewed food on the right side of my mouth for forty-six years. Imagine that.

Doc Phil told them that my jaw was trying to compensate naturally by grinding down the teeth that were causing my squinting, constipated faces, along with the tension in my jawbone. It was why I naturally chewed my food on my left side. Doc Phil started his work, demonstrating to the other dentists where the bite needed to be corrected.

The process involved about three and a half hours with mini-breaks required and many bites on different types of paper strips that Doc Phil used to calibrate his work. Starting with the left side, talk some more Greek, drill a little, then to the right side, talk some more Greek, repeat, and then back to the left side, repeat, and on and on. You will get a kick out of the Greek dentists use. Sounds like "bi-cup-silly, bisk-cally, tri" this and that. You will definitely feel like a snapping turtle. Remind you, I did not need one needle of Novocain nor major teeth work. Relief.

THIS IS ONE EXPERIENCE I WHOLLY RECOMMEND TO EVERYONE. GET THE BITE RIGHT.

The sensations that I experienced as Dr. Phil's work progressed were at times indescribable. I could notice the tension slowly draining from my jaw joints. My mouth was actually experiencing a new comfort. My whole character seemed to relax. No more tension!

My wife was amazed when I came home. I actually sat still for all that time—and in the notorious torture chair to boot. This is one experience I wholly recommend to everyone. Get the bite right. I am grateful that Doc Phil is teaching other dentists. As awareness grows, more people will be helped. I only wish that this could have happened earlier in my life.

Thanks, Doc Phil,
John H.

JANUARY OF 1988, *with my mouth locked open, I went to the emergency room. The doctor there thought my jaw was broken and wanted to admit me for a procedure. By the time the doctor got there I had my mind made up not to let them admit me. Later in the year I saw another physician and dentist who wanted to operate. I was referred to this team by a dentist who wouldn't work on my teeth unless I had this surgery first. Actually, there were three dentists who felt this way. None of these dentists knew if they could help me. I asked the doctors for names of patients who had been helped by the surgery. I spoke to one patient. She said she was in more pain than before the surgery.*

Thank God for Dr. T! What he did for me was a miracle. I haven't had any pain since. I can chew anything I want to. I used to be afraid to chew. I worried all the time that I would hurt my jaw and not be able to get my mouth open again for the rest of my life.

I have a friend who was a patient of Dr. T. She kept telling me not to do anything until I saw Dr. T. Every time I saw her, she would ask if I had called him yet, and thank God I made that call.

Dorothy B.

I FIRST MET DR. T. *in the 60s when he became our family dentist. At that time Dr. T. took care of all my general dental requirements as well as corrective work. At times I would complain that my teeth were hurting, but Dr. T. was unable to find anything wrong, and it was diagnosed as stress. When Dr. T. left El Cajon, I saw a dentist near my home for normal checkups and the periodic problem of my teeth hurting. Each time I was told nothing was wrong and that stress was probably causing the problem.*

AFTER HE MADE THE CORRECTIONS THE PAIN I HAD BEEN HAVING IN MY TEETH WAS GONE.

My mother and sister-in-law have both been helped by the occlusal correction procedure and recommended that I visit Dr. T. I went to see Dr. T. and reviewed the problems I have had for years. Dr. T. explained what occlusal correction was and gave me a booklet to read. He took impressions and X-rays and set my next appointment to review the findings. When I went for my appointment, Dr. T. explained and demonstrated on the molds exactly what was causing the problems I was experiencing. After he made the corrections the pain I had been having in my teeth was gone.

I have had a couple of tune-ups and found that when my teeth hurt it is an instant signal my bite has a problem. Since my initial correction I have not had a migraine. *Could this procedure end all my migraines for the future? What I wonder is why haven't dentists been required to learn occlusal correction to save patients from all this pain?*

Sincerely,
Sharon D.

MY MOUTH AND *jaw prior to treatment had a tendency to feel tight and under stress. At times when I was under unusual stress my jaw actually locked up on me. After my initial procedure and while I was still in the doctor's chair, my mouth and jaw felt as though a great weight had been lifted, and there was no longer any stress felt in my face by the jaw hinge. I can feel a better contact when closing my mouth, and it is easier to chew.*

Camille Z.

I COULD HAVE *written sooner but decided to wait to be sure. I think we can safely say I am 100 percent cured of TMJ. I no longer have even a flicker of pain, and I'm not restricted from any type or texture of food. This had been the case for at least five consecutive months. By the way, I've almost eliminated milk from my diet and decreased my chocolate intake from a minimum 6 oz. a day to a maximum of 3 oz. per week! Thanks for hanging in there, making me believe, and seeing me through this most difficult time.*

Sincerely,
Suzie D.

I THINK WE CAN SAFELY SAY I AM 100 PERCENT CURED OF TMJ. I NO LONGER HAVE EVEN A FLICKER OF PAIN, AND I'M NOT RESTRICTED FROM ANY TYPE OR TEXTURE OF FOOD.

I CAME TO DR. T. *in January 1984, after approximately three to four years of facial pain, headaches, weeks of sleepless nights, root canals, and an apicoectomy. In 1979 I started developing very severe headaches two to three times a day. I never got headaches, so for me this was a drastic change. I had just recently been to my dentist, so I dismissed my teeth as the problem; therefore, I called my physician, who after a thorough exam ordered a complete sinus and cranial X-ray work up which was negative for any disease process. He gave me a prescription for Tylenol with codeine—even these did not provide relief. I can still remember crying and calling UCSD at 2 A.M. to check and see how many tabs could be taken safely at one time. Even with doubling the amount, only minor relief resulted. My doctor was to have me visit a neurologist. This sounded drastic, so I felt before I took this step, I would check with my dentist once more. He took bite impressions and discovered that my wisdom teeth were throwing my bite off. After having the teeth removed, all my headaches disappeared. What a blessing! He explained that the removal of these teeth may result in a need for adjustment of other teeth. After this, I started living in his office—one to two times a week, returning for adjustments to certain teeth—my biggest complaint being I couldn't sleep at night. Whenever I shut my mouth during sleep I woke up. A root canal was finally done on the upper first bicuspid right side. This seemed to take care of the problem for a while. Sometime later, this same tooth started to keep me awake again. X-rays showed severe bone loss. I returned to the endodontist, who performed the root canal and recommended an apicoectomy.*

After the apicoectomy and bite adjustments, my whole bite was thrown off. The way I described it to my dentist was, "It feels like someone shoved a cookie sheet in my mouth on my left side." Nothing meshed on my left side. Within a few weeks after the apicoectomy, I started having trouble with the second lower molar on the left side—keeping me awake! Another root canal was done, but the tooth continued to keep me awake. My dentist tried adjustment after adjustment. At one point he asked me how many times the tooth awakened me; I said, "Anytime my teeth come together." He asked me if I could live with that. After that suggestion, I decided to seek another dentist. This pain was real. I knew something was wrong. Also, I didn't realize how badly my bite shifted until one day I went to thread a needle and none of my front teeth met.

"IT FEELS LIKE SOMEONE SHOVED A COOKIE SHEET IN MY MOUTH ON MY LEFT SIDE."

My old dentist plus a couple of friends had mentioned Dr. T.'s name. After the first appointment, I left feeling there was hope. First, he instructed me to sleep with a small cotton ball between my teeth—simple but effective. I slept! The numbness and tingling decreased. Within two weeks, he fitted me with an upper retainer and lower wire appliance. After six months with these appliances, I was fitted for braces for fine adjustment, which I wore for another six months. Shortly after their removal, Dr. T. did a bite correction. My teeth looked great, and my bite functioned beautifully, but most importantly—no more headaches or pain, and I could sleep. If a headache or facial tingling returns, a minor adjustment usually remedies it!

AFTER THE FIRST APPOINTMENT, I LEFT FEELING THERE WAS HOPE.

I AM MORE *than grateful to Dr. T. for the elimination of chronic pain and the return of dental function and to his staff for their continued support.*

Thank you,
Judy P.

BRIEF HISTORY OF MY DENTAL WORK

I am seventy years old, and my dental problems extend over a long period of time.

Childhood

During my years in elementary school I had a great number of cavities filled. During my high school years I had many of the above fillings drilled out and replaced due to new cavities next to the previous fillings. As a result—all of my back teeth have been filled since that time. Surprisingly, none of my teeth have been required to be removed as a result of these cavities.

College

During this period I had three wisdom teeth pulled. The upper two teeth were not impacted. The lower left wisdom tooth was somewhat impacted. The fourth wisdom tooth on the lower right was very badly impacted. Since it was not hurting, the tooth was not extracted. During this period I also had an upper front tooth removed and a gold bridge installed. The tooth nerve had died as a result of a blow I had received while working on a telephone pole. This event occurred approximately two years before.

After College to Present Time

After the above events my dental problems seemed to be over. I had my teeth cleaned and checked regularly, except for an occasional filling. Everything seemed to progress well.

Then about 1960 I started to notice pain in the area along my lower right jaw. It was intermittent and would last for a few minutes at a time. It seemed most noticeable after I had gone to bed. In addition to the pain I could also hear a "clicking" sound in my right ear.

The pain seemed to center at the base of my impacted tooth, and I became suspicious that it might be causing the problem. The other thing I noticed was the feeling that the impacted tooth was trying to push my other teeth out of line—especially toward the front of my mouth (right side).

As time went on, over five or six years, it became progressively worse. I asked my dentist if the impacted wisdom tooth could be causing this problem. He said no. Finally, it became so painful that I had a doctor at the oral surgery clinic remove it. He said the impacted tooth might have caused the pain since it was located very close to a nerve running along the lower jaw. Removal of the tooth seemed to help at first, and the clicking sound in my ear virtually stopped. When it did occur, it was for a very short time—usually one or two minutes. At the same time I still got the pain along the jaw and the sensation that something was still trying to push my front teeth out of line.

About 1970 I had a series of tooth enamel failures on my left side upper and lower rear teeth. As a result several gold caps were installed to protect the teeth. At the time the dentist mentioned that this was probably caused because these teeth closed and touched before the teeth on my right side. Consequently, he felt the pressure was breaking the enamel on my cavity-filled rear teeth.

About 1980 the pain in my lower right jaw continued to increase, both in frequency and the amount of pain. My dentist X-rayed the teeth but could find nothing wrong.

In the spring of 1985 he referred me to a periodontist to check my gums. X-rays and other checks failed to detect any problem. I was next referred to an endodontist for any possible nerve problems. None was discovered. His X-rays failed to show any problem. He did suggest it was possible that there might be a very small cavity, around or under one of my numerous fillings. Since there was no apparent other solution, my dentist then drilled out all the fillings on the lower right-hand side of my face. This procedure not only failed to cure the problem but actually made it much worse as I now had very sensitive teeth, plus the pain along the jaw. When the pain along the jaw started, it also made all of the nerves in the teeth just filled hurt along with it.

This seemed to trigger the pain along my jaw, and it now became more frequent and more painful.

It was difficult to describe the pain. At one time it might start near the center of my mouth and then gradually work its way to the rear. The next time it might be near the center of the right jaw and could either stay at that point or work its way toward the front or rear. The next time it might start at the rear, stay there, and finally go away. At other times the whole lower right side of my mouth would ache. In these cases the pain seemed to be in the jawbone itself.

Although each pain cycle would not last more than two or three minutes, it was extremely painful and seemed to be coming at shorter intervals and becoming more painful. Shortly thereafter my dentist referred me to a physician in La Mesa. My dentist felt there was nothing more he could do since he believed the source of the pain was not dental. He felt that it might be in the sinus or something of that type. After the physician heard my description, he mentioned it sounded like TMJ and was preparing to send me to another doctor. At that time I decided to see you. My daughter had told me three months before that it sounded like the same thing that her friend had and that it was TMJ.

MY DENTIST FELT THERE WAS NOTHING MORE HE COULD DO SINCE HE BELIEVED THE SOURCE OF THE PAIN WAS NOT DENTAL.

The rest is history. After making impressions of my teeth to correct the bite, you took the necessary steps to accomplish the correction. As a result of your very first adjustment, August 19, 1985, both the pain in my jaw and the nerve pains in my teeth vanished. Neither pain has reoccurred since. It seems like a miracle!

IT IS HARD TO BELIEVE THAT SO MANY DOCTORS CHECKED ME OVER YET FAILED TO IDENTIFY THE PROBLEM.

It is hard to believe that so many doctors checked me over yet failed to identify the problem. I have written at some length above in the hope that it may assist you to aid someone else who may find himself in the same situation.

Thanks,
Bruce L.

DEAR DR. T.,

Thank you for changing my life and making me healthy again. Less than a year ago, and before starting treatment with you, I was given some terrible facts about what I was facing in my future.

After two years of experiencing severe attacks of illness, doctors told me I had Ménière's Disease.

An untreatable, incurable disease—and I would have these attacks at any time with no warning and should expect to lose my hearing. For a woman of forty who had been in excellent health since the moment I left my mother's womb, this was a real shock.

This nightmare started about three years ago. Other than an unusual amount of headaches, I was feeling normal until one afternoon, as I was driving home, I felt light-headed and dizzy. My ear felt as if it had water in it. I was thankful that I was close to home as this condition got worse, and as I think back on it now, I don't know how I made it home and on to the couch. If I tried to get up, I would fall over. I had no balance control whatsoever. This lasted for three hours or so, and then I got up and soon felt normal again. It happened several times over the next few months. The severity and duration of these attacks were similar, until one morning as I woke up and opened my eyes, I noticed the flowers on our bedroom wallpaper were going in circles. I felt extremely dizzy; I had a high-pitched ringing in my ear; and I soon felt nauseous. I could not stand up and had to crawl to the bathroom. This condition lasted all day.

I went to the doctor and described my illness. It was then he told me of Ménière's Disease. He gave me a hearing test at that time. He explained to me that there was no medication for my problem and that if I had another attack to take a motion sickness type of medication, which might help me through the attack. He also asked me to call him after I had another attack, as he wanted to give me another hearing test.

My attacks continued over the next few months, sometimes a month or so apart, but each attack seemed to get worse. One day my physician had to come to the house to treat me as I was too ill to get up. I had been flat on my back for hours, couldn't move my eyes or any part of my body without feeling total nausea, and the loud ringing in my ears was almost deafening.

My physician made an appointment for me to see a doctor at Scripps Hospital. These tests lasted about two hours, and since they were sent to my physician, I never saw them and have no idea what the results were. Another hearing test showed I had lost some hearing in my left ear since the last test. The first hearing test, by the way, had shown I had excellent hearing in both ears. My physician said he thought I should go to the House Clinic in Los Angeles and find out if something could be done for me, as he thought I was too young to lose my hearing. I never did go because of you, Dr. T.

I came to you one day to have my teeth checked, and you suggested I consider doing something about correcting my jaw and bite as I had a TMJ problem that might cause me problems in the future. Little did we know then, those problems had begun two years earlier.

I started treatment with you on April 1, 1986. Almost overnight all the ailments I had experienced the last two years vanished. I *have not had a headache or any attacks of illness in almost a year.*

I am healthy again, Dr. T., and I owe it to you. My last hearing test that I asked to have a few months ago showed I have regained the hearing I had lost in the left ear. You have made me feel like a new person. This last year has been a wonderful and rewarding experience, and I thank you.

Sincerely,
Natalie C.

I HAVE NOT HAD A HEADACHE OR ANY ATTACKS OF ILLNESS IN ALMOST A YEAR.

AUTHOR'S NOTE: She had an excessive overjet of the upper front teeth, which violated the second principle of organic occlusion. There was no immediate anterior disclusion, forcing the bite to destroy the anatomy of all the posterior teeth and to place too much strain on the TM joints. Her treatment was orthodontics to move the anterior teeth back to a normal position.

DEAR DR. T.,

So often people aren't thanked or complimented for work they do well. I have called you the "Miracle Dentist" to so many of my family and friends, but I haven't told you. This letter is to thank you for the superior work you have done correcting my bite and easing the discomfort of TMJ. Not only has that diminished, but I am thrilled that I no longer have periodontal problems. Last, but not least, I thank you for the superb orthodontic work you performed on my son, Bradley. You are truly "The Miracle Dentist."

Sincerely,
Mary R.

DEAR DR. T.,

I am a sixty-eight-year-old male living in Los Angeles, California. I have had Type II diabetes for five years. I have been constantly in treatment for it under excellent medical care. I am not insulin-dependent, but I do depend on the following medicines: glucophage, glucotrol, actos, zocor, and privinil, all of them at their maximum dosage or close to it. I also follow the prescribed diet and exercise regime. I am relatively fit.

Prior to Dr. Taylor's bite correction in mid-February of 2009, my daily fasting blood sugar measurement was consistently running at 140 to 160 mg/dL. After Dr. Taylor's intervention the same measurements, with exactly the same diet and exercise regimes, have dropped to 99 to 120 mg/dL. The target is 117 mg/dL.

There has not been any other factor involved in the change. Therefore, the only possible conclusion is a direct relation between the bite correction and the improvement on my diabetic condition.

Sincerely,

Jack

AUTHOR'S NOTE: Jack came to me after several unsuccessful diagnoses by others. He had lived with his unusual bite for twenty-odd years, with it gradually deteriorating, until the upper left central incisor fell out due to extreme bone loss. All of the upper teeth were periodontally hopeless. I saw him and discussed various options, the first being total extraction of the remaining upper teeth. Together we decided the better option would be to cut the crowns off of all the upper teeth, leaving the roots in place to provide a stronger bone structure to support an upper denture. I pulp capped the nerves (instead of root canals) to preserve the strength of the root and placed gold thimble crowns on the remaining stumps.

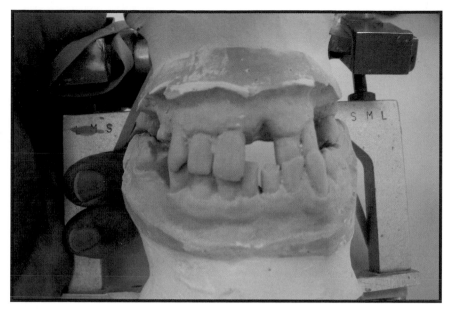

FIGURE 52: *Front view of original bite displayed on model showing crossbite on left side and drifting on the right side*

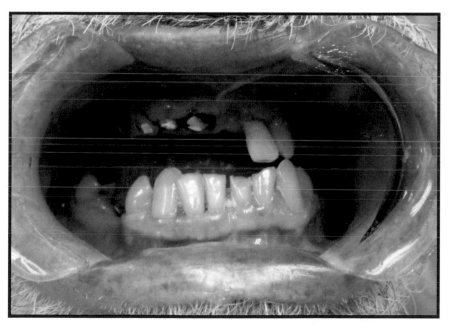

FIGURE 53: *This view shows the operation in progress, about halfway through. The stumps are pulp capped and the roots are prepared for thimble crowns. It also shows the lower jaw in centric relation, touching #11, where it slides into a crossbite.*

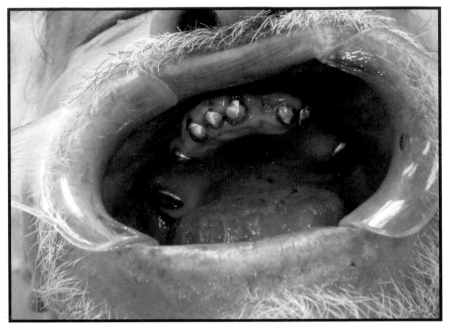

FIGURE 54: *Thimble crowns*

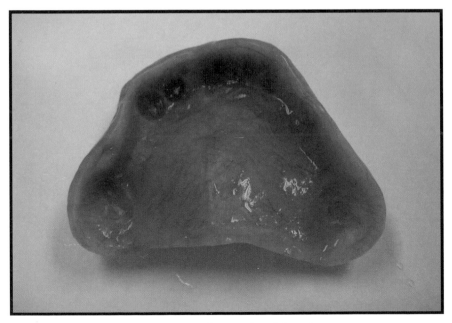

FIGURE 55: *Overdenture that fits on thimble crowns*

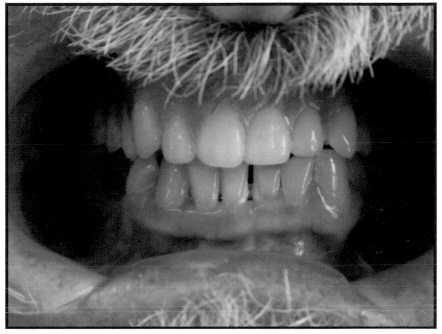

FIGURE 56: *Overdenture in place correcting to organic occlusion*

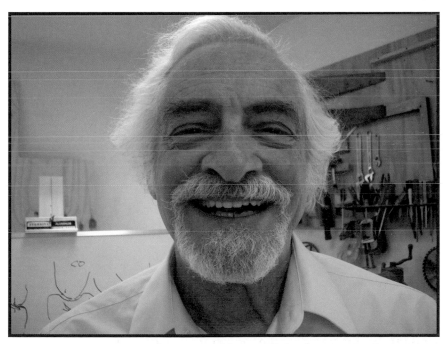

FIGURE 57: *Patient with corrected bite able to chew properly again*

NOTE TO DENTISTS: This patient's bite was so distorted that when he closed in centric relation the lower left cuspid touched outside of the point of the upper cuspid in a crossbite (see figure 53), so that when he closed down, the upper cuspid slid inside the lower cuspid, forcing his jaw forward and to the right (see figure 52). When he finally closed completely, the lower right centrals and cuspid jammed the weaker upper right incisors and cuspid, pushing them out to his right. Missing posterior teeth allowed the bite to overclose and magnify the adverse forces on the remaining front teeth, particularly the uppers. The lower teeth were periodontally much stronger than the uppers, even though he had three missing teeth, which will be replaced with implants or bridgework.

My Message to You

WHY SHOULD WE not look for a better way to practice dentistry? Why not move to a new higher plain? Our obligation to ourselves is to keep learning the new stuff. Sometimes the new stuff is not beneficial to the patient. More than likely it is more profitable to the salesmen and manufacturing companies. This is our job—to discern the difference.

In the first blush of enlightenment, we began to make bridgework to replace neglected and usually extracted teeth. Then we found out that they did that in ancient times in Egypt. In the late twentieth century we began to implant artificial stuff in the bones where teeth used to be. Now this technology is exploding with better stuff. The selection of implant fixtures is changing daily. There is a rush to find the best there is. But the interest in how the bite works is very low on the scale.

This interest (gnathology) by the dental profession really took off in the early- to mid-twentieth century. The main idea was that how the bite was engineered was more important than the other stuff. But it was competing with the war on periodontal disease. This disease was emerging as the frontrunner of how teeth were lost.

When gnathology was discovered in the mid-century, how the teeth fit together was not considered too exciting a subject. Yes, it solved all kinds of problems: periodontal problems, grinding, and the baffling TMJ problems. But gnathology seemed to take a backseat to the more exciting technology of implants. Like cell phones, computers, and HD TV, the science of putting teeth back in the mouth without ooziness of denture paste was mind-boggling.

So the rush to new stuff was now newsworthy, again pushing aside gnathology. So I believe TMJ has been relegated to a corner of dentistry that believes it is treatable. This corner has no particular way out. We can't regain the front page of the blogosphere. Our voice is too small to reshape the dental schools. We exist as a small body of pioneers who still believe that gnathology is the way to go.

When we meet together in the biannual conference of the International Academy of Gnathology, we will hear scientific sessions reporting on a variety of opinions and beliefs about gnathology.

Because the interest of those in attendance is so great, the atmosphere is charged with excitement. Not because there is total agreement among all the participants but because we agree on one thing: that gnathology does come first and is the answer to the most difficult dental problems. For example, there are two or more distinct schools of thought on the exact procedure that should be used for occlusal correction. This subject will probably not be discussed (except at my table clinic) because it would violate the dogma of Charles Stuart, DDS, one of our genius founders.

Of maybe the 98 percent of all dentists who do not practice gnathology, half do know that the bite is important and try to improve the bite with splints. The other half probably will continue with their original dental school teaching. The problem or direction of dentistry as I see it boils down to: (1) improper treatment for TMJ; (2) reinforced by literature that repeats the mistake of disbelief; and (3) little or no teaching of this "bite correction" procedure.

AFTER DOING IT WRONG FOR ALMOST THIRTY YEARS, I MADE THE RADICAL CHANGE THAT I NOW RECOMMEND TO ALL DENTISTS.

When I was teaching at USC Dental School, I wanted to teach in the department of crown and bridge. I was told that I had to take some extra courses. I had been doing crown and bridgework for about twenty-five years then, and it stunned me to think that maybe I didn't know what I was doing. Yes, I could recall a couple of bridges that had failed, but I didn't believe at the time that lack of knowledge was to blame. Boy, was I wrong. I attempted to place a bridge into the "existing" bite, which I assumed was correct. A few years later, after taking the necessary courses, I completely changed direction, and gnathology became my burning interest. I changed my delivery system from a five-chair office to a one-chair office and large dental lab, where I did all my own lab work. That was almost thirty years ago. After doing it wrong for almost thirty years, I made the radical change that I now recommend to all dentists.

First, recognize that you may not know the importance of gnathology. Second, seek to change and learn the most underutilized procedure in dentistry: occlusal correction to organic occlusion. *Make the change.* Good luck.

INDEX

Aller, Barry, 110
American Journal, 144, 146
arthrocentesis, 125
arthroscopy, 74–75
articular disc, 15, 17
articular tubercle, 15
articulators, 75, 83–85, 90, 108, 112
  Stuart, 99, 103, 105, 113–14, 124
  Whipmix, 80–81, 91, 124
Austin, Art, 110

Benson, James, 110
bicuspid extraction practice, 32, 142
bite
  accuracy, 116
  correction, 12–14, 27, 30, 60, 61, 75, 116, 120–21, 125, 127–28, 129, 145, 153, 156, 159–60, 167
  evenness, 53, 128, 147
  problems, 8

  stability, 52, 138
  transitional, 118
bonding, 94–95, 129–130
braces, 139, 142–43, 153
bridgework, 21, 32, 51, 164–65
Brocket, Sheldon, 112
bruxism, 49–51, 97–99
Burzynski, Stanislaw, 61

Cal Tech, 12
Carville, James, 9
cavities, 154–55
centric relation, 29, 32, 34, 41–42, 49, 52, 59, 63–64, 84–85, 87, 112–13, 118, 121–22, 131, 134, 162, 164
Cheraskin, Emanuel
  "The Arithmetic of Disease," 29
chewing muscles, 54, 69, 71, 120
Chiang Kai-chek, 107
Chinnaut, Claire Lee, 107
City Heat, 134
Clinton, Bill, 9

ABOUT THE AUTHOR

PHILIP L. TAYLOR, DDS, has been practicing dentistry in California since 1950.
During the 1970s, while teaching at the
USC School of Dentistry, his practice was
revolutionized when he learned the principles of gnathology from his mentor Dr.
Gus Swab. Now, after working according to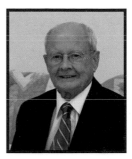
these principles for decades and witnessing the results, Dr. Tay-
lor is a tireless advocate for bite correction as the solution to
the many problems associated with TMJ.